Sincerely,

YOUR
GYNECOLOGIST

Jeff,

Sincerely,

YOUR
GYNECOLOGIST

We are still in the business.

NGOZI OSUAGWU, MD, FACOG

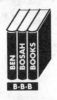

BEN BOSAH BOOKS
B·B·B

For information regarding permission, write to:
Ben Bosah Books, PO Box 671, New Albany, Ohio 43054

Publisher's Cataloging-In-Publication Data

Names: Osuagwu, Ngozi, author.

Title: Sincerely, your gynecologist / Ngozi Osuagwu, MD, FACOG.

Description: New Albany, Ohio : Ben Bosah Books, 2022. | Includes bibliographical
references and index.

Identifiers: ISBN 9780996908474 (hardback) | ISBN 9780996908481 (ebook)

Subjects: LCSH: Gynecology--Popular works. | Obstetrics--Popular works. | Women--
Health and hygiene. | Self-care, Health. | LCGFT: Didactic fiction.

Classification: LCC RG121 .O752 2022 (print) | LCC RG121 (ebook) | DDC 618.1--dc23

Library of Congress Control Number: 2021946313

Photo: Shellee Davis

Cover Art: Paschal Anyaso

Cover and Book Design: Zakirunissa Karthigeyan

For more information about Ngozi Osuagwu, MD, FACOG
visit www.ngoziosuagwumd.com.
For more information about the book, visit www.benbosahbooks.com

For my Children,

Chiedu,

Chidi and Chinenye

DISCLAIMER

While most of the information in this book is about medical issues, it is not medical advice and should not be treated as such. The material in this book is only informational in nature, and meant to facilitate conversations with your healthcare providers. Although written by a licensed medical doctor, it is not meant as a substitute for the advice of, and care by your licensed medical professional. The letters in this book are based on the author's experience, but no references have been made to any person nor should any be inferred. All the names are used fictitiously. The author and publisher disclaim any liability arising directly or indirectly from the use of this book.

Throughout the text, links to websites are provided. These sites were carefully screened and included correct information at the time of review; however, it is important to remember that the Internet is a dynamic entity—websites and the information posted within them are constantly changing and evolving. The information contained within these sites are not intended for diagnostic purposes, nor is it intended to replace the consultation of your own doctor or licensed medical practitioner. The author and publisher make no representation or warranty regarding the accuracy, reliability, completeness, currentness, or timeliness of the content, text or graphics. The links provided to these websites are for information only — they do not constitute endorsements of the sites.

The information provided on the websites mentioned in this book should not be used during any medical emergency or for the diagnosis or treatment of any medical condition. A licensed physician should be consulted for diagnosis and treatment of any and all medical conditions. Call 911 for all medical emergencies. The author and publisher cannot be responsible for any incorrect information or medical decisions made on the basis of information contained within any of these websites.

ACKNOWLEGEMENT

I f anyone told me that it would take sixteen years to do a sequel to the American edition of Letters to My Sisters: Plain Truths and Straightforward Advice from a Gynecologist, I would have stared at them in disbelief. But it has been that long. It was a long time ago, and a lot has changed in medicine and women's health. In that time, I have grown as a doctor and a human being, which is a good thing because the experiences make this book a more seasoned one.

In the intervening time, I have toiled at this manuscript, cheered on by the many people who enjoyed my first book and conveyed to me how my voice and writing style led to their improved well-being and that of those who hold their affection. I have stuck to that same style of addressing medical and health-related issues in this same blunt style, now tempered more with love and compassion. I hope that you find this latest book equally useful.

This book is in your hands because of the time and selfless efforts of many people. The quality of this book was enhanced significantly because of their input. I cannot thank them enough. I want to thank Janice Brillson, Dominique Delma, Karen Drake, Marilu Faber, Alyssa Kujawa, Ruby Kyles, Maggie Lin, Cara Blessley Lowe, Jason Melillo, Wendy Neal, Chinwe Osuagwu, Beverly Owusu, Sandra Quick, Dara Richardson-Heron, Chinyere Tobias, and Taylor Wilkinson.

Armed with galleys of the book, the individuals mentioned above read and provided valuable comments that were essential to the quality of the final book. My gratitude knows no bounds to this legion of pre-readers.

My long-time copy editor, Kim Lundy, took the raw manuscript and put me through the grinder with her comments and queries. Addressing her comments and queries significantly improved the readability of this book. Zakirunissa Kartigeyan handled the book and cover design and did a bang-up job. After so many iterations and ideas, the minimalistic painting of Paschal Anyaso would be the selected art for the cover. Mamta Jha created the book's index. The author's photograph is by Shellee Davis. I thank every one of these aforementioned people profusely.

My patients equally deserve credit for this book. My desire to be a better doctor for them is the primary motivator for the books I write, and the meditations on how to better serve them are the root of my inspiration. I hope this book becomes an extension of my dedication to serving their healthcare needs.

Even with the best effort and intention, my family remains the rock behind me. My mother, Grace Osuagwu, my children, Chiedu, Chidi, Chinenye, and their father and my husband, Chukwuemeka were my biggest cheerleaders even as they offered constructive criticisms. I love you and thank all of you for the sacrifices you make by giving me the space and time to indulge in this activity that is also a balm to my soul.

PREFACE

This book was scheduled to come out in 2020 and then COVID hit. I wondered if this book still had relevance. I realized that COVID or not, we still have other ailments and health concerns. Sexually transmitted infections are not going away because of COVID, nor are high blood pressure, menopause, or pregnancy. What COVID has reminded me is that we cannot ignore our health. What I know from decades of personal experience and what COVID has taught me is we should prevent the diseases we can and try to optimize our health to be able to deal with those ailments that do occur.

We have had time to reset. My hope is this book gets us communicating. I am hoping we will all communicate better with our healthcare providers. I am hoping as women we will be able to communicate with each other. I am hoping there will be an increase in intergenerational communication. This is not an exhaustive book of all medical conditions that affect women. It is, however, a reflection of the common problems I see.

I have grown as a physician since my last book. I am not as brash. I truly love what I do. I love my patients, many of whom have become like sisters to me. Recently, I have been called "Dr. Mom." It is truly a reflection that I am getting older. My patients give me a reason to wake up in the morning; they give me purpose. I am thankful to God for the ability to serve in this fashion.

Sincerely, Your Gynecologist

Since the last book, I blog weekly. I continue to meditate, but I am not as diligent in journaling. I still exercise and have maintained a healthy weight. I pray that each of you stays healthy and finds purpose and happiness in your life. Please continue to share the information you find here as best as you see fit.

CONTENTS

Content

REVISITING THE PATH TO GOOD HEALTH

Dear Zoe,

Thank you for reaching out to me. It has been 16 years since I last wrote to you about charting your own path to good health. After you reached out, I reread the letter I sent you back then.

I hope the last 16 years have been good to you and you are doing well. I am still employed and do not believe I will ever go back to solo practice. It is so hard to be an obstetrician/gynecologist and do it alone. The trend now is to have physicians employed by large health care systems. I am fortunate, I have been able to practice the way I have always wanted: putting the patients at the center. It is funny how that has become so important, but we knew about it over 16 years ago. That was one of the reasons you decided to see me at the time. I still see my patients as my sisters.

I am older now and realized I have to double down on self-care and would encourage all of us to do the same. We cannot take care of others without taking care of ourselves. Self-care is not selfish; it is self-less. It is important to give of our healthy selves to take care of others.

I still believe in having a routine. I wake up and pray each morning. The Almighty is an important part of my life. The Almighty is at my core. I then get up, scrape my tongue, brush my teeth, and exercise. There are several components of exercise—aerobic, resistance, flexibility, and balance. I make sure to incorporate each into my weekly routine. Afterward, I meditate and then take my shower. Sometimes, I meditate prior to exercising. It really depends on my mood. Meditation is definitely a must each day. Taking time each day to be present and focus on just breathing is a wonderful experience.

As I mentioned to you in the last letter, breakfast is important to me. I no longer eat on the go. I sit down to eat my breakfast. I sit down to eat all my meals. I pack my lunch most of the time except on special occasions. My dinner is in the early evening. I love my fruits and vegetables.

Sleep has become extremely important to me. Everything I read emphasizes how important sleep is to maintaining good health. I have learned how to use the "do not disturb" setting on my phone. There is nothing that important that cannot wait until the morning. There are five people in my life who can bypass that setting and they know how important it is for me to sleep. Sleeping can be difficult especially when on call covering the physicians in my group. Babies come when they want, and not between 9 a.m. and 5 p.m, as would be our preference if we had the choice. I still get those 2 a.m. deliveries and while one day I will have to leave those deliveries to the younger physicians, today is not the day. I still love delivering babies.

I have been truly blessed with a great family and know everyone is not so fortunate. For the most part, I have also benefitted from having an excellent work family and some of my best relationships are with those who are not blood relatives. Loneliness is a serious risk factor for all types of health diseases, and it is so important we develop a circle of people that have our backs. I am happy to have the blood relatives and people like you I can call my sisters. Being part of the community through church, book clubs, sororities—the list can go on and on—is good for our health.

Do I cheat once in a while with my routine? Of course; no one is perfect. But I then get back to my routine without judgment, not feeling guilty, because I am human. Routine has been helpful. It can change depending on what I read; I make adjustments depending on what I learn.

Thanks once again for reaching out to me to find out how I was doing and for encouraging me to finish this book. I hope it will not take another 16 years to correspond again.

Take care,

Ngozi

TEENAGE QUESTIONS

Dear Aisha,

heard from your mother you are now feeling better. By now, you should be nearly finished with the antibiotics I prescribed for the urinary tract infection. While you no longer have lower belly pain, burning while you urinate, and the urge to use the bathroom all the time, it is important you finish all of your medicine.

I was troubled you felt too uncomfortable to ask me some of the questions you and your friends had put together to ask a physician. Your mother suggested you might have been too embarrassed to share them with me. You should never feel embarrassed to ask me any question, especially when it comes to health. Doctors like you to ask questions. My daughter, who is about your age is constantly asking me questions.

Before I answer the questions, I want you to know I use "you" not because my response is actually addressing you, but because it is easier for me to answer the question that way. I know it is not necessarily "you" asking, but some of your friends. Here are the answers to the questions you sent:

Can you get pregnant the first time you have sex?

Yes, it is possible to get pregnant the first time you have sex. In fact, most girls who get pregnant the first time they have sex do so because they do not think they can get pregnant that easily. Each time a girl has sex and does not use birth control, there is a chance she can become pregnant. If the plan is not to become pregnant, then birth control must be used all the time. What confuses many people is that there might be times you have sex without birth control and don't get pregnant. This all has to do with ovulation, when an egg is released from your ovary. The way you become pregnant is when the egg meets the sperm. For teenage girls, it is not easy to predict exactly when you are going to ovulate so that you can avoid having sex during that time. Having sex without birth control is very risky because one day you will get pregnant. The take-home message is this: If you decide to have sex and the plan is not to get pregnant, you must *always* use birth control, even if it is your first time.

Which one is safer: oral sex or vaginal sex?

Oral sex and vaginal sex—and let us add anal sex (or "butt" sex)—are about the same. None is safer than the others. You can get a sexually transmitted disease whether you are having oral, vaginal, or anal sex. The only way you can get pregnant is with vaginal sex, but you can get any of the sexually transmitted diseases having oral, vaginal, and anal sex. With butt sex, you can get it even faster. You can get chlamydia, gonorrhea, herpes, syphilis, human immunodeficiency virus (HIV), human papillomavirus (HPV) —you name it; you can get it. If you are going to have any type of sex, you should use protection. For oral sex, the boy can put on a condom and the girl can take another condom and cut it to cover the entrance to the vagina, called the vulva. The goal is to have a barrier between the mouth and the penis or the vulva. For vaginal and anal sex, a condom should be used. While on this topic, I think it is important for every girl to inspect the boy's penis before it enters the mouth, the vagina, or the butt. This means you have to turn on the light. I know some girls have told me this is disgusting, but if it is that the case, it should not be entering you. If you notice any blisters, cuts, or discharge, do not let it enter you. The take-home message is neither oral nor vaginal sex is safer, and you should *inspect* anything that is going to enter your body, including a penis.

Are you still a virgin if you use a tampon or see a gynecologist?

You are still a virgin if you use a tampon or see a gynecologist. You lose your virginity when you have a penis enter your vagina. Tampons are convenient, especially since you are young and involved in sports, so feel free to use them. Make sure you change the tampon as directed on the package. You should not have a tampon in the vagina for more than six hours. I think it is also a good idea not to use a tampon overnight. If a tampon is left in the vagina for a long time, it can cause a serious infection. As for gynecological exams, these days, when teenagers come to a gynecologist, the gynecologist may not have to perform a pelvic exam, meaning that nothing would enter your vagina during the visit. It all depends on the reason they are seeing the gynecologist. At any rate, a doctor's exam will not affect your virginity. The take-home message for you here is that the only way to lose your virginity is if a penis enters the vagina.

When do you know that you are gay?

For me, I must admit this is a difficult question to answer. I imagine it is difficult for anyone to pinpoint an actual age at which you know you are gay. I am going to take it from a girl's perspective. As a girl, you will have friends who are girls and friends who are boys. When we reach puberty, our sex hormone levels change, and we begin to have thoughts and desires. Sometimes we become attracted to girls and sometimes we become attracted to boys. There comes a point in our lives, usually in our later teenage years the attraction is extremely powerful, and we realize we are interested in someone of the same or of the opposite sex. It is probably at that time you know. However, I cannot determine an age—some people realize it later and some earlier, but everyone eventually figures it out. However, at your age it is normal to have a best friend that is a girl, and you can be jealous, and she can hurt your feelings, and that does not make you gay. It is okay to not like the hottest fashion and prefer to hang out with boys, and that also does not make you gay. It is okay to say no to a guy who might want to have sex with you if you are not ready or do not wish to have sex, and that does not make you gay. The take-home message is eventually most people figure out whether they would rather be with someone of the same or of the opposite sex for the rest of their lives. If anyone feels confused, it is a good idea for them to talk with an adult they trust who would be supportive, and most of the time that adult happens to be a parent.

I must admit these questions were interesting. I am glad you and your friends are spending time having these discussions. I am always available to come to your school and speak with you and your classmates if you have any more questions, but if you prefer to send written questions, I am always happy to respond this way as well.

Take care,

Ngozi Osuagwu, MD, FACOG

SEXUAL RELATIONSHIPS AMONG ADOLESCENTS

Among sexually active high school students, 7% had sexual intercourse for the first time before age 13 years.[1]

27.4% of high school students reported being sexually active.[1]

Nearly 46 % of sexually active high school students did not use condoms the last time they had sex.[1]

Vaginal intercourse or oral sex is more common than anal sex with a partner of a different sex.[2]

Sources: [1] Szucs LE, Lowry R, Fasula AM, et al. Condom and Contraceptive Use Among Sexually Active High School Students – Youth Risk Behavior Survey, United States, 2019. MMWR Suppl 2020;69(Suppl-1):11–18. DOI: http://dx.doi.org/10.15585/mmwr.su6901a2 (Accessed February 16, 2022)

[2] Lindberg LD, Firestein L, Beavin C. Trends in U.S. adolescent sexual behavior and contraceptive use, 2006-2019. Contracept X. 2021;3:100064. Published 2021 Apr 8. doi:10.1016/j.conx.2021.100064 (Accessed February 16, 2022)

TEENAGER WITH AN ABNORMAL MENSTRUAL CYCLE

Dear Abena,

Your mother wanted me to write to you because she wanted you to see me in my office. She told me you are afraid of having a pelvic exam and some of your friends told you the pelvic exam was very uncomfortable and even painful. Your mother is very concerned because she says it seems as if you are always on your period and there are times you have had to miss school because of your period. She said when you were in middle school it was not that bad, but now you are in high school, it is difficult for you to maintain your grades since you are missing so many days of school.

Let me be very clear: you are 16 years old, and I do not plan to perform a pelvic exam. I rarely perform pelvic exams on 16-year-olds—I can count on one hand how many I have had to do this in the past year. The purpose for your visit is to see what we can do about your periods. We have to make sure you do not have a serious medical problem causing you to have periods that are associated with severe cramps preventing you from going to school.

A normal menstrual cycle is every 21 to 45 days. A cycle goes from the first day of one period to the first day of the next period. The first day of your period is Day # 1 of your cycle. If you record each time your period starts, I can show you how to evaluate a menstrual cycle. Your period should not last more than 7 days. If it is lasting more than 7 days, this is not normal, and we need to find out what is happening. If you are wearing pads and/or tampons and you are constantly having accidents where you are staining your clothing or bedsheets, this is not normal. We will need to find out why you are having heavy bleeding. Some girls have cramps with their period, which should get better with nonsteroidal anti-inflammatory drugs (NSAIDs) such as ibuprofen. You can buy NSAIDs without a prescription with your mom's help. Some girls need a stronger medication which requires a doctor's prescription. Sometimes we have to give young girls hormones, such as birth control pills. The reason we do this is not that the young girls are having sex, but rather these pills shut down the ovaries so the ovaries do not produce chemicals that can cause cramps.

I cannot treat you over the telephone. I would need to see you and speak with you to figure out what is happening. I would like your mother to come with you because she can help with your family history and might help you with your medical history, especially when you were a baby.

What I would like you to do is start writing down when your periods start and whether the bleeding is heavy or light. I would like you to also describe how you feel; for example, are the cramps so bad you are unable to go to school? Some girls find it is easier to download a menstrual calendar app to their cell phone and record the information so that it is always available. For now, you can ask your mother to give you ibuprofen to help alleviate your cramps. My best advice is to start the ibuprofen the minute you see blood and use it as directed on the bottle for at least two days. There is no need to wait for the pain if you know you experience it with your period.

If you decide you want to see me, tell your Mom and she will schedule an appointment. I look forward to seeing you soon.

Take care,

Ngozi Osuagwu, MD, FACOG

NORMAL MENSTRUAL CYCLES IN ADOLESCENT GIRLS

Menarche* (median age):	12.43 years
Mean cycle interval:	32.2 days in first gynecologic year
Menstrual cycle interval:	21–45 days is typical
Menstrual flow length:	7 days or less
Menstrual product use:	3–6 pads or tampons per day

*Menarche – start of your menstrual cycle.

Source: American College of Obstetrician and Gynecologists. Menstruation in Girls and Adolescents: Using the Menstrual Cycle as a Vital Sign, Committee Opinion No. 651. Obstet Gynecol 2015;126:e143–e146.

CHLAMYDIA: EXPEDITED PARTNER TREATMENT (EPT)

Dear Paula,

I needed to write this letter because I am not sure if you clearly understood what I was saying when you were in the office. You appeared distracted when you were here, and I wanted to find another way to explain what was happening.

You are 18 years old and have been dating Michael for three years. You have told me on several occasions he is your first and only boyfriend and you began having sex with him about a year ago. In that time, you have tested positive for chlamydia twice.

Chlamydia is a sexually transmitted infection, which means you get the infection through having sex. You do not get it from a toilet seat or sharing towels; you get it by having sex. You told me you never had sex until last year. When you came to the office about two years ago, I checked you for chlamydia and it was negative. I also placed the implant in your arm for birth control. At that time, I made it clear to you although the implant was great in preventing pregnancy, it would not protect you against sexually transmitted infections. I told you it was important to use condoms to protect against sexually transmitted infections. You can use the implant and condoms.

When you tested positive for chlamydia about one year ago, I treated you and asked you to come back to the office four months later to be retested. You could not wait four months, so you came back after two months, and I rechecked you and your test came back negative. You said you did not have sex with Michael during that time. You also told me Michael told you he had no symptoms and did not think he needed to be treated. The fact is you do not have to have symptoms to test positive for a sexually transmitted infection.

Remember, you did not have symptoms when you tested positive for chlamydia the first time. Michael should have been treated then. There is a process called expedited partner treatment (EPT), in which a doctor can write a prescription for both their patient and their partner without requiring the partner to be examined. There are rules that must be followed to do this and not all pharmacies offer this service, so you might need to call first. Whether or not you use this process, Michael needs to be treated. He needs to know that this is important.

You came to me this time because you had an abnormal vaginal discharge. You tested positive for chlamydia again. I can treat you repeatedly, but you will continue to test positive for chlamydia as long as you continue to have sex with Michael while he remains untreated. You also have to know that chlamydia, if not treated in a timely manner, can cause a more serious infection that could lead to problems getting pregnant in the future.

Paula, you need to talk to Michael because he needs to be treated. If he does not have a doctor, he can go to an urgent care, the emergency room, or the health department. If he is reluctant to see a doctor himself, I can send the prescription for him under EPT. It does not matter whether or not he has symptoms; he needs to be treated. After you take the medication, you should not have sex with him until he is treated. If you have chlamydia, he has chlamydia. I do not know what Michael is doing or not doing when it comes to having sex with other people. It could be when he met you, he did not know he had chlamydia. All I want is for him to get treated.

Since it is sexually transmitted, anyone he has had sex with before you should be treated. I want to remind you how important it is to use condoms. Although it cannot guarantee that you will not get chlamydia, it is much better than not using anything.

If you have any questions or want to talk more about the contents of this letter, please call the office to discuss further, or schedule an appointment to see me. Hopefully, you have already taken all your medication.

Sincerely,

Ngozi Osuagwu, MD, FACOG

FACTS ABOUT CHLAMYDIA

Chlamydia is the most commonly reported sexually transmitted infection in the United States, with more than 1.8 million cases reported in 2019. Approximately one-third of cases among women were reported from private physician offices. Its prevalence is highest among adolescents and young adults aged 15–24 years old.

Chlamydia infections in women can lead to serious consequences including pelvic inflammatory disease (PID), difficulty becoming pregnant, ectopic pregnancy (pregnancy not in the uterus), and chronic pelvic pain.

Chlamydia is transmitted through sexual contact with the penis, vagina, mouth, or anus of an infected partner.

Chlamydia can be transmitted from an untreated mother to her baby during childbirth.

Chlamydia is known as a "silent" infection because most infected people are asymptomatic (without symptoms) and do not have abnormal physical exams.

Yearly screening of all sexually active women younger than age 25 years old is recommended.

Source:

Center for Disease Control and Prevention. Reported STDs in the United States, 2019. https://www.cdc.gov/nchhstp/news-room/docs/factsheets/std-trends-508.pdf (Accessed June 19, 2021)

Workowski KA, Bachmann LH, Chan PA, et al. Sexually Transmitted Infections Treatment Guidelines, 2021. MMWR Recomm Rep 2021;70(No. RR-4):1–187. DOI: http://dx.doi.org/10.15585/mmwr.rr7004a1 (Accessed February 16, 2022)

Sincerely, Your Gynecologist

LONG-ACTING REVERSIBLE CONTRACEPTIVES

Dear Tanya,

It appeared you were a little confused when you left the office. First, let me say I am happy you decided to come and see me. You are now 18 years old and will be leaving to go to college. I know, when you saw me today, your plan was to get on the pill. Birth·control pills are a good contraceptive option. Along with preventing pregnancy, they provide other non-contraceptive benefits. Birth control pills help decrease menstrual cramps and decrease the amount of blood flow during your period. This means they can make your periods lighter. They have also been shown to decrease your risk of getting ovarian and endometrial cancer. There are birth control pills that allow you to have your period once a month or once every three months. My concern is you mentioned you were not sure you would be able to remember to take a pill every day and you need to take a pill every day for birth control pills to work. This is why I mentioned "LARCs."

LARCs stands for long-acting reversible contraceptives. These are birth control methods that really do not require you to do much. You do not have to worry about missing a pill; the only thing you have to do is come into the office to get it placed. When I talk about LARCs, I am talking about intrauterine devices (IUDs) and the implant that is placed in your arm. Although LARCs can last 3–12 years, you do not have to keep it in that long. I know I gave you some information to take home when you were in the office.

There are several types of IUDs; however, they can be broken down into two types: IUDs that contain hormones and the IUD that does not contain hormones. The IUDs that contain hormones can last from 3–7 years. The IUD that does not contain hormones contains copper and lasts for 12 years. The primary way that an IUD works is by creating a hostile environment in the uterus, where the IUD is placed, and killing the sperm before it reaches the egg. Hormonal IUDs also make your cervical mucus thick to stop the sperm and thin out the lining of the uterus so your menstrual flow is light. The IUD with hormones can make your periods irregular, and in some cases stop your periods altogether. The IUD that contains copper can cause your periods to be heavy, but they will be regular.

The other LARC is a small rod we place under the skin in your arm. We call it an implant. It has hormones. Although the package says it last for three years, it has been shown to work for up to five years. It can cause irregular and unpredictable bleeding, and for some women it can stop their periods all together. It works by preventing ovulation, meaning you do not release an egg. If you do not release an egg, the egg cannot meet the sperm and be fertilized. The hormone in the implant also thickens the cervical mucus like the IUD which contains hormones.

There are possible side effects when you use hormonal birth control, such as nausea, breast swelling, and abdominal bloating, but most of the symptoms go away with time. There are complications that can occur when placing the IUD or implant, but those complications are rare. The major one is uterine perforation (going through the uterus) when placing the IUD. One thing you should know is when I am placing an IUD, I do not use any force. This may help decrease the risk of perforation.

You also should keep in mind LARCs prevent pregnancy. LARCs do not protect against sexually transmitted infections. You will need to use condoms.

Please read the information I provided to you. I am really proud of you for having such insight on what you can and cannot do. If you cannot take a pill every day and you do not want to become pregnant, then birth control pills are not for you. Please schedule an appointment to place any of the LARCs as soon as possible. Ideally, I would like you to be on your period, within the first five days. Just call the office when your period starts and we will have you come in within that time frame.

Sincerely,

Ngozi Osuagwu, MD, FACOG

STATEMENTS ON THE USE OF LARCS FOR ADOLESCENT PATIENTS

American College of Obstetricians and Gynecologists (ACOG)

 "Long-acting reversible contraceptives (LARC) have higher efficacy, higher continuation rates, and higher satisfaction rates compared with short-acting contraceptives among adolescents who choose to use them."[1]

American Academy of Pediatrics (AAP)

 "Pediatricians should be able to educate adolescent patients about LARC methods including the progestin implant and IUDs. Given the efficacy, safety, and ease of use, LARC methods should be considered first-line contraceptive choices for adolescents."[2]

Sources: [1]American College of Obstetricians and Gynecologists. Adolescents and Long-Acting Reversible Contraception: Implants and Intrauterine Devices. Committee Opinion No. 735. Obstet Gynecol. 2018 May;131(5):e130-e139. https://www.acog.org/-/media/project/acog/acogorg/clinical/files/committee-opinion/articles/2018/05/adolescents-and-long-acting-reversible-contraception-implants-and-intrauterine-devices.pdf (Accessed January 3, 2018); [2]American Academy of Pediatrics, Committee on Adolescents. Contraception for Adolescents. Pediatrics 2014;134(4):e1244–e1256. http://pediatrics.aappublications.org/content/pediatrics/134/4/e1244.full.pdf (Accessed June 19, 2021).

ADVICE FOR COLLEGE

Dear Chichi,

Congratulations! Your mother told me you decided to go to The Ohio State University. I am so proud of you. Unfortunately, I will not be able to attend your party, but I will be there for the graduation ceremony. I am writing to you not only as your doctor, but also as your godmother. I looked at so many graduation cards and could not find one that really expressed how I feel or provided the advice that I want to give you. As you know, my daughter is also graduating. Her graduation is one week after yours. I have been thinking about what advice I wish to give her as well and decided to write a letter to both of you. Although there is so much to say, I have condensed it down to 12 guiding principles. I just want you to realize your parents and I were once teenagers. We went to college. We know you have to go through your journey, but we would like the road to be less bumpy.

1. **Put God first.** I believe there is a higher power who we can rely on. Do not forget to pray.

2. **Trust your instincts.** We all have some little bug inside of us telling us when we should or should not do something. Some call it our gut feelings. Some say it is the Holy Spirit talking within us. I ask that you listen to your gut. There are times your friends might want you to do something and you just do not feel it is right. DO NOT DO IT! A rule of thumb is once you put on your pajamas for the night, the only reason you should go out is for a life-or-death situation.

3. **Do not drink alcohol, smoke cigarettes, or take street drugs.** I just want to remind you that the legal age to drink alcohol is 21 years. It can really wait until then. You can have fun without alcohol, and you will actually remember what happened. Cigarettes and drugs are addictive. Still, you will be offered all three. Some will even say that you are too smart to get addicted. Your response should be, "I am too smart to start." DO NOT BE AFRAID TO SAY NO. It is okay to be called a goody two shoes. If the people around you are your true friends, they will not pressure you to take anything or do something that is potentially dangerous.

4. **Never leave your drink unattended.** If you did not open the drink yourself, if you did not see how the drink was made, or if your drink was open and left unattended, throw it away. It is not worth taking the drink. People do put drugs in drinks. Carry your own water bottle in your bag; this way you will always have a drink.

5. **While driving, never text, and always wear your seatbelt.** Regarding texting, never text as a driver, and limit the texting even when you are a passenger. You always need to be aware of your surroundings. As for the seatbelt, you should always use it, whether you are a driver or a passenger.

6. **When you do decide to have sex, make sure it is on your terms, and please use condoms.** Ideally, I would love for you to wait until you are married, but I am a realist. Remember, you would not be here if your parents did not have sex. I have children, so clearly, I have had sex. I know the thought might seem appalling to you, but we are all sexual beings. You will have guys coming to you and telling you all sorts of things like if you really care for me, you would have sex with me. Remember when you decide to have sex, it should not be to prove you love someone, it should be because you have found someone who cares for you and because you care for them. That person should be someone who wants you to be your best and is willing to be with you even if you are not ready to have sex. Also, before you do anything, both of you should get tested for

human immunodeficiency virus (HIV) and other sexually trans-mitted infections. Do not be afraid to ask the person whether they have had anything in the past and also ask how they feel about their mother. If they love their mother, they will treat you well. USE CONDOMS. If the condom breaks, there is emergen-cy contraception that you can use within 72 hours of the acci-dent. You need to finish school before starting a family. Smile. I have known you all your life and know at this point in your life, you are not ready to be a parent.

7. **Eat your fruits and vegetables daily.** No one will be there to police the type of foods you are eating. Along with your daily vitamins, I would like you to remember to add fruits and vege-tables. They contain antioxidants and macro- and micronutri-ents to help you stay healthy.

8. **Eat breakfast.** This is the most important meal of the day. It helps with brain health and really makes you sharper academ-ically.

9. **Do not be a couch potato.** Even though I know you do not plan to be on a sports team, you still need to exercise regularly. The "Freshman 15" is a reality, and we can help combat this weight gain by exercising regularly.

10. **Always remember you are in college for the education, but be open to the experience.** If you are like my daughter, you have just been focusing on the college experience. You need to remember that your parents are sending you to school to get a good education. We want you to graduate as happy and in-dependent individuals—and I would stress independent. How-ever, college is amazing. You will meet different people and be exposed to so many things. Embrace all of the differences and be willing to learn. Embrace your community on and off cam-pus. Join a club. Learn something new. You might not know this, but I actually was part of the drama club and performed in plays in college, yet I never was in theater in high school. Be adventurous and explore.

11. **Look in the mirror every day and know you are a wonderful gift from God**. You have a purpose in this world. You are beautiful and you are loved. Spend at least five minutes a day embracing this fact. When times get rough in school, do not give up; ask for help. Know that you were meant to be where you are and you can overcome all obstacles.

12. **Listen to your parents, most importantly your mother.** You need to remember your mother loves you. She will never give you bad advice. She wants the best for you. Always go to her with any questions. She is guaranteed to have your back.

I love you and I am so proud of you. Peace, love, and happiness always.

Your Godmother,

Ngozi Osuagwu, MD, FACOG

WHY GO TO COLLEGE?

1. **Higher Earnings -**There is a strong correlation between education and wages, and those with higher degrees often out-earn those who skipped college.

2. **Increased Job Security -** Graduating with a college degree typically leads to more job security, which means you are less likely to face unemployment. This is especially true when there is a downturn in the economy.

3. **Greater Life Satisfaction -** More schooling could lead to a happier life—people with bachelor's degrees tend to be happier than those without one. College grads also tend to have longer marriages than those with a high school education, and better marital outcomes can lead to increased happiness.

4. **Easier Access to Health Insurance and Other Benefits -** College graduates are more likely to work for companies that offer health insurance benefits than high school grads. College graduates are also more likely to have access to other perks like paid vacation and sick days, stock options, student loan assistance, and retirement plans.

5. **Better Health Outcomes -** Having a college education can actually help you live longer. There are many reasons that higher education correlates with better health. Those with college degrees have greater access to health insurance, which can lead to more preventative screenings. The higher salaries that often accompany college degrees can also lead to safer housing,

better access to healthy foods, less exposure to pollutants and greater access to green spaces.

6. **Opportunity to Pursue Niche Interests** - College can also be a place to pursue new passions and expand your worldview. You can learn new skills.

7. **Expand Your Professional Network** - You have access to people who can impact your professional standing including how much you earn. You will have access to people in your industry. Most importantly you have access to the college's alumni network.

Kumok, Z. & Hahn, A. (2022, February 7), 7 Compelling reasons why you should go to college. Forbes Advisor. https://www.forbes.com/advisor/student-loans/why-should-you-go-to-college/ (Accessed February 27, 2022)

HUMAN PAPILLOMAVIRUS VACCINE

Dear Ms. Tsosie,

It was a pleasure to meet you and your daughter at your recent appointment. I know you were reluctant to have me prescribe any hormonal medication to help your daughter with her menstrual cramps. As I mentioned during your office visit, the best thing to do is to make sure she starts taking ibuprofen the minute she sees blood. We know she gets menstrual cramps, so there is no need to wait until they begin. She will need to take the ibuprofen as prescribed for at least the first two days of her period, even if she stops having pain. After the first two days of her period, she can then take it as needed.

I am also writing for another reason. I asked whether she had received the human papillomavirus (HPV) vaccine and you mentioned you did not want to discuss it. You mentioned that your daughter was not having sex and you did not think she needed the vaccine. You also mentioned you were not sure if the vaccine was safe because it is new. I know I sent you home with information, but I wanted to tell you a little more about the vaccine from my perspective. I got the sense you did not want me to have the conversation in front of your daughter, and that is why I decided to write.

The HPV vaccine has been around since 2006. It is a safe vaccine. All three of my children have received it. I believe it is safe. Will there be side effects? It is hard to say. Two of my children completed the series without a problem; however, my youngest did not because she developed an allergic reaction to the first shot and was advised not to continue.

The best time to get the vaccine is before you become sexually active. We want to make sure the person receiving it has not already been exposed to the virus. HPV is the most common sexually transmitted infection. The chances of getting the virus are high once you have sex. Although the vaccine can be given between the ages of 9 and 45 years, we like to give it to children in middle school, between the ages 11 and 13 years. We can still give the vaccine if someone has had sex or even if they have tested positive for HPV; however, the vaccine is most effective before one starts having sex.

There are many types of HPV, and they can be classified into two groups: those that are high risk and those that are low risk. The high-risk types put you at risk for cancer, particularly cervical, anal, and oral cancer. The low-risk type is usually associated with genital warts. We now have the vaccine that protects against nine different HPVs. The vaccine particularly protects against HPV 16 and 18, which are the cause of 70 percent of cervical cancers. The vaccine also protects against HPV 6 and 11, which are the low-risk types and are associated with 90 percent of the genital warts. The vaccine can also be given to boys.

I think you should reconsider your stance against having your daughter vaccinated. If you have any questions, please do not hesitate to contact the office. I look forward to hearing from you soon.

Sincerely,

Ngozi Osuagwu, MD, FACOG

FACTS ABOUT HUMAN PAPILLOMA VIRUS

HPV is the most common sexually transmitted disease in the United States. Fourteen million people become infected with HPV every year. Seventy-nine million people who are infected with HPV are in their late teens and early twenties. Nineteen thousand cancers in women every year are caused by HPV. About 12,000 cancers in men every year are caused by HPV. The cancers include cancer of the cervix, vulva, vagina, penis, and anus. It is also associated with cancer in the back of the throat, including the base of the tongue and tonsils (called oropharyngeal cancer).

Source: Centers for Disease Control and Prevention. Genital HPV Infection – CDC Fact Sheet. https://www.cdc.gov/std/hpv/HPV-FS-July-2017.pdf (Accessed June 22, 2021).

BI-CURIOUS

Dear Deidra,

Please forgive me. Unfortunately, I do not have a poker face, and I hope that my expression did not give you the wrong impression. I have no problems with your sexuality, I had just never heard of one referring to themselves as "bi-curious." That term is new to me. Usually, I hear people call themselves lesbian, bisexual, or gay. I am learning. The reason I asked about your sexuality was to be able to order the appropriate tests and to give you some advice on staying healthy.

You are now 21 years old, so I did perform a Pap smear. If your Pap smear comes back negative, your next Pap smear will be due in three years. You still need to see me every year for an exam. Since you have had sex with a man within the past year, I also tested you for gonorrhea and chlamydia. It is recommended that you get checked for gonorrhea and chlamydia regularly if you are younger than 25. You mentioned you have been exclusively with women for the past two months and did not want to discuss birth control. However, I think you should be aware of what is available since you disclosed you still have an interest in dating men. I have enclosed information on the various types of birth control in case you choose to consider it.

You should also be aware being with a woman does not eliminate the risk of sexually transmitted infections (STIs), so you should still practice safe sex. You can still get STIs. For example, if your partner has a herpes sore on her mouth and you engage in oral sex, you might end up with ulcers in the vulva area. Please consider asking the proper questions like whether they have a history of STI, whether they have been with a person of the opposite sex or whether they are exclusively with you. Use dental dams for oral sex. As always, if you are using any toys, please make sure that you wash them with soap and water and dry them properly. I have had patients with recurrent vaginitis due to not cleaning their toys well.

Finally, you mentioned you are not sure how long you will be with your girlfriend—and you still have feelings for your ex-boyfriend and might still be in love with him. I think it is important to be honest with yourself and your girlfriend. I think you should discuss your feelings about your ex-boyfriend and that you are not ready for a serious relationship. You do not want to hurt her feelings if she is interested in a long-term relationship and you are not.

If you have any questions or concerns, please do not hesitate to contact the office. Also, please sign up on the patient portal so I can email your results.

Sincerely,

Ngozi Osuagwu, MD, FACOG

WHAT AM I?

Bi-curious characterized by an openness to or curiosity about having sexual relations with a person whose sex differs from that of one's usual sexual partners, curious about exploring or experimenting with bisexuality

Heterosexual of, relating to, or characterized by a tendency to direct sexual desire toward someone of the opposite sex

Homosexual of, relating to, or characterized by a tendency to direct sexual desire toward another person of the same sex

Lesbian of or relating to homosexuality between females

Gay homosexual between males

Bisexual of, relating to, or characterized by sexual or romantic attraction to members of both sexes; engaging in sexual activity with partners of more than one gender

Transgender of, relating to, or being a person whose gender identity differs from the sex the person had or was identified as having at birth; especially of, relating to, or being a person whose gender identity is opposite the sex the person had or was identified as having at birth

Queer sexually attracted to members of the same sex; differing in some way from what is usual or normal

LGBTQ lesbian, gay, bisexual, transgender, and queer; lesbian, gay, bisexual, transgender, and questioning (one's sexual identity)

Source: "bi-curious," "heterosexual," "homosexual," "lesbian," "gay," "bisexual," "transgender," "queer," and "LGBTQ." Merriam-Webster.com. https://www.merriam-webster.com (Accessed January 13, 2018).

TELL HER THAT YOU LOVE HER

Dear Ms. Smith,

You asked me to see your daughter today because you feel she is out of control. You mentioned she has a boyfriend whom you dislike and that you were worried that she might be having sex and wanted her to get on some sort of birth control. You also told me you did not think she was capable of remembering to take the pills, so you wanted her to use something like the shot. I understand that you could not make the appointment today because you were at work. Thank you for sending the note giving us permission to see her without you. I am writing to share information from her visit and she is aware I am writing this letter to you and wanted me to share this information with you.

You have a wonderful daughter. She is bright and full of energy. She wants to finish school and understands that education is important, but her world is so different at school. She mentioned she has never heard you tell her you love her. She also told me you complain about her weight and you hate that she refuses to perm her hair. Her boyfriend, on the other hand, tells her repeatedly he loves her. She realizes he may not be perfect but believes that he loves her. She told me that they have had sex, but they always use condoms. She is not interested in getting pregnant and has decided to use the implant. I was able to place the subdermal implant in her today. I reminded her that it does not protect against sexually transmitted infections and she would still need to use condoms.

Your daughter is an astute child. She understands it is hard to be a single mother and it has been difficult for you to make ends meet. She worries that you blame her for her father's death—if he had not gone out to pick her up that fateful night, maybe he would still be alive. She needs you. She needs a mother. She wants to talk with you. She told me you are always tired. I urge you to make time to talk with her, listen to her, and tell her you love her. She wants and needs support, especially at this time in her life, and not just from her boyfriend or school friends, but from you, her mother.

I believe both of you would benefit from family counseling. I would be glad to make that referral with your consent. If there is anything else I can do, please do not hesitate to call me.

Sincerely,

Ngozi Osuagwu, MD, FACOG

Mama

Mama, Mama

I need your help

I need you to show me some direction

I need you to tell me that I am special

I need you to show me the way

Mama, Mama

Don't let me go

Hold me please

BEING A MOTHER

Dear. Ms. Massie,

I admitted your daughter to the hospital because she is experiencing pelvic pain, but in reality, it is mostly due to social issues. It did not make sense that your 15-year-old child has not been in school for the past two weeks. During our discussion you told me you have lost total control and cannot force her to go to school. If you as a mother does not have control over your 15-year-old, who should? Also, I am concerned about her health. About a year ago she was treated for chlamydia and now she has been having pelvic pain for the past three days.

Being a mother is hard work however, at the end of the day, you are her mother and must bear some responsibility. Your daughter did not ask to be born. She came into this world with the expectation that some adult would guide her. That adult has to be you, Ms. Massie—her mother. It cannot be her teacher. It cannot be her pediatrician. It cannot be her boyfriend. It must be you.

I have been thinking about the comment you made about no longer having control. She is 15 years old and if you cannot control her, who should? The police? The state? I have known you for a long time. When do you think you lost control? Was it when she was two years old and you allowed her to call you by your first name because you were buddies, or was it when she was five years old and you were bringing in your boyfriends? Maybe it was at 10 years old, when you allowed her to try your cigarettes or when she was in middle school and you allowed her to hang out with her friends, without a curfew or any adult supervision.

It really is okay to say no to your child. It is okay for your child to hate you because you have rules. Children really want rules. She does not need a friend in you; she needs a mother.

I admitted her to the hospital for pelvic inflammatory disease, but I will also be calling the social worker. The social worker can provide resources. I think both of you need counseling. I have tried to make referrals in the past and you refused. It is not too late to be the mother that she needs. Please work with the social worker. I thought by writing this note and handing it to you, you might decide to make some changes and get some help.

Sincerely,

Ngozi Osuagwu, MD, FACOG

MISCARRIAGE

Dear Ms. Barry,

I deliberately chose not to say much today while you and your daughter were in the office. I thought it was important for us, as adults, to be on the same page when we were talking with your daughter. Your daughter has what is called a missed abortion. The ultrasound a few weeks ago showed a fetus that was alive, and at that time she was eight weeks pregnant. You informed me she recently had some bleeding and cramping while she was in gym class. The ultrasound today showed a fetus that only measured 10 weeks' size with no heartbeat. She should have been 12 weeks by this time. She is having a miscarriage. The medical term is missed abortion.

It is important for you to understand that her gym class did not cause this to happen. Miscarriages are very common. For every five people that get pregnant, one person will have a miscarriage. There is nothing anyone could have done to prevent this.

At this time, she has several options. The first is to do nothing. Eventually she should bleed and pass the pregnancy. I cannot predict how long that process will take. The second option is to give her medicine that will help start the expulsion process. She would take this medicine at home. She will have a lot of cramping and eventually pass what is in the uterus. The major complication that can occur with this method is bleeding, and she could end up needing surgery. The third option is for me to take your daughter to the operating room and remove what is in the uterus surgically. The name of the surgery is a dilatation and curettage, or D & C. Although this is a very safe procedure, there are risks to all surgeries. The risks for D & C include bleeding, infection, and damage to nearby organs. When we are performing this type of surgery, it is possible for the instrument to go through the wall of the uterus. This is called perforation, and although it is very rare, if it occurs there can be a risk of hurting other organs like the bladder or bowels. I think the best option for your daughter emotionally would be to have the surgery.

I was writing this letter because you were interested in finding out why she had the miscarriage, but also—most importantly—because you were hesitant to discuss birth control. In terms of why she had the miscarriage, I do not know, and I am not going to perform an extensive work-up at this time to find out. Because miscarriages are so common, and at times we cannot find a cause, we typically do not order lab work to find out why it occurred until a patient has had at least three. Sometimes we can start the work-up after two miscarriages if the patient is older.

Ms. Barry, your daughter Carly is having sex, and although she has sworn up and down she would not have sex again, I think it is important we really consider having her use some form of birth control. When you told me you found out your daughter was pregnant, you were shocked and asked God to help you. You may or may not think of this as help. I think we have a wonderful opportunity to educate Carly. Both of you really need to think about birth control. She might benefit from birth control that she does not have to deal with daily. I think you need to consider one of the long-acting reversible contraceptives (LARCs). This could be the implant we put in the arm or an intrauterine device. These types of birth control last 3–12 years depending on what type she chooses. I have enclosed a brochure on each type.

I look forward to hearing from you soon; I know you and your daughter are scheduled to come back next week. If you would like your daughter to try the medication, I can call that into your pharmacy. If you want your daughter to have the surgery, let my nurse know so that we can schedule your daughter as soon as possible. If she has any increase in her bleeding, more than a menstrual flow, please call the office. Take care.

Sincerely,

Ngozi Osuagwu, MD, FACOG

WHAT IS UNINTENDED PREGNANCY?

An **unintended** pregnancy is one that was either mistimed or unwanted. If a woman did not want to become pregnant at the time the pregnancy occurred but did want to become pregnant at some point in the future, the pregnancy is considered **mistimed**. If a woman did not want to become pregnant then or at any time in the future, the pregnancy is considered **unwanted**.1

An **intended** pregnancy is one that was desired at the time it occurred or sooner. When calculating unintended pregnancy rates, women who were indifferent about becoming pregnant are counted with women who had intended pregnancies, so that the unintended pregnancy rate only includes pregnancies that are unambiguously unintended.1

Births resulting from unintended pregnancies are referred to as unplanned, and those resulting from intended pregnancies are planned.1

Less than half (45%) of the pregnancies in the United States are unintended. Unintended pregnancy is highest among poor and low-income women, women aged 18–24, cohabiting women, and minority women.[1]

Those who have an unintended pregnancy (unplanned) tend to have inadequate or delayed initiation of prenatal care, to smoke or drink during pregnancy, and to have premature and low-birth-weight infants and are less likely to breastfeed. The children of women who have unplanned pregnancies are at increased risk of physical and mental health problems.[2]

Sources: [1]Guttmacher Institute. Unintended Pregnancy in the United States. Fact Sheet January 2019. https://www.guttmacher.org/pubs/FB-Unintended-Pregnancy-US.html. (Accessed January 15, 2018);

[2]Finer LB and Zolna MR. Declines in Unintended Pregnancy in the United States, 2008–2011. N Engl J Med 2016;374(9):843–852.

DOMESTIC VIOLENCE

Dear Nikki,

This is a difficult letter to write, but I feel I have no choice. First, I want to say that I am sincerely sorry for your loss. I know Carmen was a good friend of yours. Her death was tragic, but I encourage you to use this time to pause and consider your current relationship.

My sister always says we have been missing the point when we talk to young people. We focus on sex and the use of condoms and when to say no. We focus on the prevention of sexually transmitted infections, especially HIV infection. She says it is important to have sex education, but it is equally important to talk about love education: What does love look like?

Your friend Carmen thought she was in love and her boyfriend loved her. She thought it was love because he did not want her to talk to anyone but him. Occasionally, she could hang out with her girlfriends, but she was not allowed to talk with any guy without his permission. He wanted to be her only one. Oh yes, he bought her a lot of things; I know she never lacked for anything. I know he was always saying how much he loved her. If he could not have her, no one could. He wanted to be her sole provider. When she thought about going to college, he did not understand why, since he was providing everything. He felt that there was nothing college could provide that he could not. He was her main man, and I believe she thought she was his main girl.

Now look what happened. When she tried to end the relationship, he went crazy. She tried to get a restraining order, and I believe she did, but that did not prevent him from shooting her and then killing himself. Two young lives were wasted. Nikki, is this what love looks like?

I write because you have told me in the past your boyfriend has hit you, but he really did not mean to do it. He hit you because he was upset, and you just happened to be around. You tell me he loves you, but every time you ace your exam at school, he is never happy with your accomplishments. When you needed a car to travel to one of your chess tournaments, you could not find him, so you had to forfeit the game. You did not want to take a chance and get into another person's car for fear that he would think that you were cheating on him. You rarely go out with your girlfriends. He even has you pitted against your parents. Every night he calls you and says he loves you, but is that really love?

Nikki, for me, I would rather have a man who never says he loves me but whose actions speak in such a way the whole world knows he loves me. I want someone who tries his best to make me the best person I can be and not feel threatened. I want someone who loves my family as much as he loves his family. I want someone who does not mind me getting compliments from people, because he is confident and knows he has the best. I want someone who, when he is angry, does not use me as a punching bag but can resolve his issues without violence. I want someone who also understands we might grow apart for whatever reason and that it is okay.

I am your physician, not your parent. My primary focus is your physical health, but we both know there is a powerful connection between physical and emotional health. I want to be clear with you; I am not telling or asking you to break up with your boyfriend. I am asking you to use Carmen's death as a wakeup call. A call that is asking you the following question: What does love look like?

You are not due to see me until next year; however, if you need to be seen earlier or just want to talk, please call the office. Take care.

Sincerely,

Ngozi Osuagwu, MD, FACOG

FACTS ABOUT DOMESTIC VIOLENCE[1]

Domestic violence is the leading cause of injury to women—more than car accidents, mugging, and rapes combined.

Around the world, at least one in every three women has been beaten, coerced into sex, or otherwise abused during her lifetime. Most often, the abuser is a member of her own family.

Nearly one in five teenage girls who have been in a relationship said a boyfriend threatened violence or self-harm if presented with a breakup.

Every nine seconds in the United States, a woman is assaulted or beaten.

Every day in the United States, more than three women are murdered by their husbands or boyfriends.

Help for Victims of Domestic Violence[2]

Anonymous and confidential help is available 24 hours a day through the National Domestic Violence Hotline: 1-800-799-SAFE (7233), 1-800-782-3224 (TTY), Text "START" to 88788; victims who are in immediate danger should call 9-1-1.

Sources: [1]Domestic Violence Statistics. www.domesticviolencestatistics.org/domestic-violence-statistics (Accessed July 10, 2021);

[2]National Coalition Against Domestic Violence. www.ncadv.org/get-help (Accessed July 10, 2021).

SEXUALLY TRANSMITTED INFECTIONS

Dear Ms. Mabry,

I know you are upset that during your visit I screened you for a sexually transmitted infection, but it truly was a mistake. Typically, the CDC recommends we screen all young ladies who are sexually active under the age of 25. It does not distinguish between those who are married and those who are not. Usually, I tell all my patients what tests I am obtaining, but if you remember, I had already taken a sample before you told me you did not want to be screened. I forgot to throw away the sample and my medical assistant sent it in error.

In a way, I am glad the mistake occurred, because you tested positive for chlamydia. What a lot of women do not realize is that you can be positive for a sexually transmitted infection without having symptoms. Chlamydia is the most common sexually transmitted infection, and both you and your partner will need to be treated.

My office sent your prescription electronically to your pharmacy. Please have your husband see his physician to get treated as well. I would advise you not to have sex until both of you are treated.

Obviously, there is more to this story, especially if both of you believe you are in a monogamous relationship. I believe both of you really need to talk, because others might need to be treated so this disease does not spread. If you have any questions, please do not hesitate to contact the office.

Sincerely,

Ngozi Osuagwu, MD, FACOG

FACTS ABOUT SEXUALLY TRANSMITTED INFECTIONS

Sexually transmitted infections (STIs) remain common and costly to nation's (United States) health.

Approximately one in five adults (20% of the United States population) had an STI on any given day in 2018. This is nearly 68 million infections.

STIs acquired in 2018 cost the American healthcare system nearly $16 billion in direct medical cost alone.

Nearly half (45.5%) of all new STIs in the United States occur among young people (ages 15 – 24).

Many STIs go undetected because people do not have symptoms.

Even if you have no symptoms, you can still have serious health consequences like chronic pelvic pain, life-threatening ectopic pregnancy (pregnancy not in the uterus), and infertility (difficulty becoming pregnant) if not treated for an STI.

For all individuals who are sexually active—particularly young people—STI screening and prompt treatment (if infected) are critical to protect a person's health and prevent transmission to others.

Source: Centers for Disease Control and Prevention. Incidence, Prevalence, and Cost of Sexually Transmitted Infections in the United States. CDC Fact Sheet, January 2021. https://www.cdc.gov/nchhstp/newsroom/docs/factsheets/2018-STI-incidence-prevalence-factsheet.pdf (Accessed July 10, 2021).

SEXUALLY TRANSMITTED DISEASE TESTING

Dear Ms. Dalton,

As I mentioned to you in the office, I could not test you for every sexually transmitted infection. There are over 25 types of sexually transmitted infections. So as I have done in the past, I checked you for the most common types. I can test you for these infections; however, I do not have a test for trust. This was the fourth time in the past year that you requested testing and you are still with the same partner. When you came in, you did not have any symptoms. I know that you do not have to have symptoms to test positive. I wanted to review your results.

In the office, I looked under the microscope and did not see any evidence of a yeast infection or bacterial vaginosis. I know these are not sexually transmitted but wanted to remind you I checked for vaginitis. Your gonorrhea, chlamydia, and trichomoniasis test came back negative. Hepatitis B surface antigen, hepatitis C antibody, syphilis antibody, and HIV tests were also negative. Since you did not have any symptoms for herpes, I only performed the blood test. I did not test you for herpes simplex virus (HSV) 1 antibody because you tested positive for this antibody in the past. Remember I told you that this HSV 1 is not necessarily sexually transmitted. It is a very common virus, usually associated with cold sores on the mouth; however, if you have oral sex and you have a cold sore, you can spread HSV 1 to the genital area. The HSV 2 antibody test was negative. We do not have a blood test for the human papilloma-virus (HPV). We usually check for HPV with your Pap smear once you turn 30 years old. If the test comes back negative and you have not had an abnormal Pap smear, it is not repeated for another 3–5 years. You are 25 years old and your Pap smear last year was neg-ative. Some doctors have started to check only for HPV once you turn 25 years old instead of the Pap smear. In your case, I just per-formed a Pap smear.

Our records show you have not received the HPV vaccine. Although the best time to receive the vaccine is before you become sexually active, I think it is a good idea for you to get it now.

Again, I know it is probably none of my business regarding your relationship, but I am concerned when you have been with a man for about one year and during that time you have requested tests for sexually transmitted infections four times. If you need to be con-stantly checking, maybe it is time to reflect on this relationship. Typically, most women check themselves before they enter a rela-tionship and probably at the end of a relationship. I am happy you did not test positive for any STIs at this time, but you might need to consider using condoms. It is the only method other than absti-nence to decrease the risk of getting an infection. I look forward to seeing you for your well woman visit in six months. Take care.

Sincerely,

Ngozi Osuagwu, MD, FACOG

Abstaining from sex, reducing the number of sexual partners, consistently and correctly using condoms, getting vaccinated, talking with your partner and getting tested are all effective ways to prevent STIs.

Source: Centers for Disease Control and Prevention. The lowdown on how to prevent sexually transmitted diseases. https://www.cdc.gov/std/prevention/lowdown/the_lowdown_infographic_poster_30x20.pdf (Accessed August 18, 2021).

THREATENED ABORTION (MISCARRIAGE)

Dear Ms. Martinez,

I thought it was important that I write to you because the nurse told me that you have called the office several times and are extremely anxious about this pregnancy. As I mentioned at the office appointment, bleeding during pregnancy does not necessarily mean you will have a miscarriage. I know you were upset because the physician you saw in the emergency room (ER) said you had a threatened abortion and you cannot get that word "abortion" out of your mind. You were also upset because I did not perform an ultrasound the last time you were here to make sure everything was okay with your pregnancy. I did check the heartbeat with the Doppler machine and the heartbeat was normal at 145 beats per minute.

Ms. Martinez, when I last saw you, you had been in the ER two days earlier and had an ultrasound while you were there that showed a fetus that was alive and measuring 12 weeks pregnant. The ER mentioned to you there was a subchorionic bleed, and that would explain the blood you saw. They told you, you had a threatened abortion and should follow up with me, which you did.

Let me explain again what it means to have a threatened abortion. Any bleeding in pregnancy is considered a threatened abortion, meaning that there is a chance you might have a miscarriage.

Most pregnancies will continue and result in a baby; however, there are some that might end up with a miscarriage. It is hard to know what will happen with each pregnancy, but it is always a good thing when we perform an ultrasound and see an active baby. A subchorionic bleed represents an area where the placenta separates from the uterus and the area bleeds and sometimes clots over, and that is what we are seeing on ultrasound. As the pregnancy progresses, the clot resolves and you will not be able to see the clot on ultrasound. There is absolutely nothing anyone can do and performing several ultrasounds will not change anything.

You have been my patient for 10 years, and I know how difficult it was for you to get pregnant. I sincerely want you to have a healthy baby, and I know you and your husband are willing to do anything to help ensure you do. However, bedrest, stopping work, and not having sex will not make a difference and will not change what happens at this stage of the pregnancy. I have enclosed a note for your employer ordering you to be off work for the next two weeks because I know this is emotionally draining.

I look forward to seeing you next week to see how you are doing. If you have any increase in bleeding or experience severe abdominal cramps, please do not hesitate to contact the office.

Sincerely,

Ngozi Osuagwu, MD, FACOG

Early pregnancy loss is common, occurring in 10% of all clinically recognized pregnancies.[1]

Approximately 80% of all cases of pregnancy loss occur within the first trimester.[2]

The presence of subchorionic bleeding around the gestational sac does not have a significant association with miscarriage.[2]

Sources: [1]American College of Obstetricians and Gynecologists. Early Pregnancy Loss. Practice Bulletin No. 200. Obstet Gynecol 2018;132:e197–e207;

[2]Stamatopoulos N, Lu C, Infante F, et al. Does the Presence of Subchorionic Haematoma Increase the Risk of Miscarriage? Ultrasound Obstet Gynecol 2013;42:54.

NO-SHOW

Dear Marissa,

I wanted to send a note to you before you receive the official certified letter from the office manager. Unfortunately, I will no longer be able to see you in my private office. You have been a no-show for four visits. Our policy is to send a letter of dismissal after three no-shows, but I made an exception because I have known you for many years. You have been my patient since I moved to Ohio, and that is why I did not want you to get the certified letter without hearing from me.

I mentioned to you when I gave up my former practice and decided to move to this new one, things would change. I know there was a lot of flexibility in my other practice, but I am not sure that was a good thing. Today, no one wants to wait. We no longer double book. When you have an appointment, it is your appointment time. When you do not show or when you call the office less than 24 hours ahead of time to reschedule, I have no one else to put in your slot. If I do not have anyone to put in the slot, that means I do not get paid, and my staff does not get paid. In the past, I have double booked, but patients get annoyed with the waiting time.

You mentioned you have had similar problems at the pediatrician's office as well. I know life has not been easy for you. I recognize you are a single mom with three children and juggling everyone's schedule and trying to make ends meet is not easy. You might consider establishing care with a family doctor. The advantage is they see adults and children, and then all of you will be able to see the same doctor. You have to realize if you schedule an appointment for you and the children and you do not show up, that is a large amount of time the doctor set aside for you and your family and they probably would not give you another appointment. You may consider going to a doctor who has early morning hours, evening hours, or Saturday hours. This might be easier with your work schedule.

I know transportation has been a problem in the past. You might be able to find someone on your bus route, so that if your car breaks down, you have another way of getting to the office.

The certified letter you receive will provide a number to call to help you find another doctor. You can also call your insurance company to get help choosing a new physician. They can help you find a doctor who accepts your insurance.

I know it can be difficult to get an appointment with a new family doctor and sometimes you will be told the next appointment is in three months. Take the appointment time offered, because you are at least three months closer to the appointment date than if you do not take it. Once you have an appointment, one trick for possibly getting in sooner is to call when the weather is bad and ask if there are any cancellations; if so, they may be able to fit you in since you have already scheduled an appointment.

Marissa, it is important you and your family establish care with a physician. If you need any assistance, I am available to help. Take care.

Sincerely,

Ngozi Osuagwu, MD, FACOG

SCHEDULING TERMINOLOGY

No-show – Scheduling an appointment with your healthcare provider and not showing up for the scheduled appointment without notifying the provider's office.

Rescheduling – Scheduling an appointment with your healthcare provider and then calling the office at least 24 hours before the appointment to change the appointment time.

Cancellation – Scheduling an appointment with your healthcare provider and calling the office before the scheduled appointment to state that you will no longer be coming to the appointment. You do not reschedule another appointment.

Late for an appointment – Not showing up until after the designated start time of your scheduled appointment.

Office policy – Every office has their own, unique policies on how they handle certain situations. It is important to familiarize yourself with these. An example of a policy is how an office might handle no-show appointments. They may charge you for a no-show appointment before you can be rescheduled for another appointment.

CONTRACEPTION

Dear Vanessa,

You have mentioned in the past you had no intention of becoming pregnant until you finish college and get your dream job, so I hope you understand why I was somewhat puzzled by some of your answers during your annual examination today. You mentioned you hoped you would not become pregnant. When I asked whether you were sexually active, you answered yes, but when I asked you whether you were using birth control, you said no. I then asked how you can be having sex without using birth control and not want to become pregnant. You said sometimes your boyfriend pulls out. I hope you realize "hope" and "pull and pray" are not very effective methods of preventing pregnancy. If you truly do not want to become pregnant, you really need to consider birth control methods that are known to be effective.

Birth control can be divided into two categories: those with hormones and those without. Those with hormones contain estrogen and progestin or just progestin. They can enter your body through various ways—by mouth, through the skin, or through the vagina. These include birth control pills, the patch, the subdermal implant (placed under the skin of your arm), the ring (placed in your vagina), intrauterine devices, and the shot. Besides preventing pregnancy, there are several advantages to being on birth control that contains hormones. Birth control that contains hormones can decrease your menstrual flow so your periods are lighter. They can help with menstrual cramps. They can also decrease the risk of ovarian and endometrial cancer. The major downside is birth control methods with hormones do not protect against sexually transmitted infections.

Birth control methods that do not have hormones include condoms (male and female), nonhormonal intrauterine devices, the sponge, diaphragms, cervical caps, the withdrawal method (before he ejaculates, which is pretty hard for young guys), and periodic abstinence (natural family planning method or rhythm method). Condoms and the diaphragm may help decrease the risk of sexually transmitted infections.

Another option that is not often discussed is abstinence meaning that you do not engage in intercourse. It is 100 percent effective in preventing pregnancy. There are many ways to be intimate without the penis entering the vagina.

Vanessa, none of the methods I mentioned (except for abstinence) can prevent pregnancy 100 percent of the time, but they are much more effective than "hope" and "pull and pray." I am hoping you will decide which form of birth control will work for you and pull your weight to get an appointment as soon as possible and pray that we can do this before you become pregnant.

Also, I recommend you begin taking folic acid. Folic acid helps decrease the risk of having a child with neural tube defects—problems with the brain and spine of the baby. You need to have folic acid on board early because the brain and spine of the baby usually are formed by the time one is four weeks pregnant. The amount of folic acid necessary to decrease the risk of having a child with a neural tube defect is 400 mcg or 0.4 mg per day. This can be found in multivitamins that are specific for women. If you have any questions on anything I discussed in this letter, please do not hesitate to call the office and schedule an appointment so we can talk.

Take care,

Ngozi Osuagwu, MD, FACOG

Couples who do not use any method of contraception have approximately an 85% chance of experiencing a pregnancy over the course of a year.[1]

The average number of children U.S. adults think is ideal is 2.7. To achieve this family size, a sexually active woman must use contraceptives for roughly three decades.[1]

Among contraceptive users aged 15–49 in 2018, female permanent contraception was the most common method used (28%), followed by pills (21%), male condoms and IUDs (both 13%). The two most popular methods (permanent contraception and pills) have remained so since 1982.[2]

Sources: [1]*Guttmacher Institute. Contraceptive Use in the United States. Fact Sheet May 2021. https://www.guttmacher.org/fact-sheet/contraceptive-use-united-states (Accessed August 18, 2021).*

[2]*Guttmacher Institute. Contraceptive Use in the United States. Fact Sheet May 2021. https://www.guttmacher.org/fact-sheet/contraceptive-method-use-united-states (Accessed August 18, 2021)*

EMERGENCY CONTRACEPTION

Dear Marcy,

Enclosed is a prescription for the pills to be used for emergency contraception. Although you are at an age where you can walk into to the pharmacy with a valid photo ID and get them without a prescription, it is much cheaper if you have a prescription and you have insurance.

As we discussed, the only reason I am informing you about emergency contraception is that you were adamant about finishing college and graduate school before having a baby. You stated you do not want to use any birth control that contains hormones, and you were not interested in the nonhormonal copper IUD. I am happy you are using condoms all the time; however, condoms are not very reliable in terms of preventing pregnancy. Accidents do occur, and when they occur, emergency contraception is the backup. Regardless of whether you were using birth control with or without hormones, I would still recommend you use condoms. Condoms are excellent for reducing your risk of sexually transmitted infections.

Emergency contraceptive pills work by delaying ovulation. It does not cause an abortion, and if you are already pregnant when you use it, it will not harm the unborn child. For emergency contraception to work effectively, you need it to use it within 72 hours of the condom accident. Some people have used emergency contraception as many as five days after the accident, but it is less effective after 72 hours. Also, you should know the copper IUD can be used as a form of emergency contraception, and you can then keep it in to help prevent future pregnancies.

Because it works by delaying ovulation, you really need to continue using condoms or abstain from sex until your next period if you are not interested in having a baby. Also, your period might be irregular, meaning it may not come when it was due to come after using the emergency contraceptive pills. If your period does not begin within two weeks of using the pills, please perform a pregnancy test.

I know you stated you had not heard about emergency contraception and you would share the information with your friends at school. Some of your friends may think of using it as a form of birth control. It is not a reliable form of birth control. It should not be used as a "Monday-morning-after-having-fun-all-weekend pill."

Please remember to sign on to the electronic patient portal website with your secure code. This will make it easier for us to communicate while you are in school. When I receive the results from the gonorrhea and chlamydia test, you will be able to see the results through the portal. Have a wonderful semester. I look forward to seeing you next year for your well woman exam.

Take care,

Ngozi Osuagwu, MD, FACOG

Emergency contraception is a therapy used to prevent pregnancy after an unprotected or inadequately protected act of sexual intercourse. Several forms are available:

Formulation	Timing if Used After Unprotected Sexual Intercourse	Access
One tablet, containing 30 mg of ulipristal acetate*	Up to 5 days	Requires a prescription
One tablet, containing 1.5 mg of levonorgestrel†	Up to 3 days	Available over the counter without age restriction
Two tablets, each containing 0.75 mg of levonorgestrel	Up to 3 days	Available over the counter to those 17 years and older with photo identification
Combined progestin–estrogen pills (birth control pills)	Up to 5 days	Requires a prescription
Copper IUD‡	Up to 5 days	Requires an office visit and insertion by the clinician

*Ulipristal acetate is more effective than the levonorgestrel-only regimen and maintains efficacy for up to 5 days.

†The levonorgestrel-only regimen for emergency contraception is more effective than the combined hormonal regimen and is associated with less nausea and vomiting.

‡Insertion of a copper IUD is the most effective method of emergency contraception.

Source: Practice Bulletin No. 152: Emergency Contraception. Obstet Gynecol. 2015 Sep;126(3):e1-e11. doi: 10.1097/AOG.0000000000001047. PMID: 26287787. https://www.acog.org/clinical/clinical-guidance/practice-bulletin/articles/2015/09/emergency-contraception (Accessed August 18, 2021)

NONHORMONAL CONTRACEPTION

Dear Rachel,

You cannot do the same thing over and over and expect different results. There is no such thing as an "oops" baby. When you are having sex and not using birth control, you will get pregnant. It might not happen tomorrow or the next month, but one day it will happen. You are 27 years old and unmarried and have three children with three different men, and now you are pregnant with number four. I truly do not know what you want me to tell you.

When you came to see me last year, you told me you had found "the one." You told me this guy was different. You were in love. I was truly happy for you. You told me you had been trying to have a baby with him over the past year, but nothing was happening. I thought maybe you would see this as a sign from God. This man might be your one and only, but he already has two children and is not taking care of either of them. I wondered why you would think he would want to take care of his child with you; if he was in love, he should be able to love the three you already have.

I am not sure why I am writing. It may not be important. After all, you are pregnant, and we can only move forward. I guess I am writing because we really need to consider what we are going to do after this baby comes. What birth control will you use? There are many options available, and you really need to consider all of them.

I know that you are not interested in anything with hormones. We have the copper IUD that does not have any hormones, and no, it does not cause abortions. The way it works is by creating a hostile environment in the uterus so that the sperm dies before meeting the egg. The copper IUD is effective for 12 years, but if you desire to remove the IUD before that time, we can.

You can also consider the diaphragm. The only catch is you must be an active participant—the diaphragm only works if you use it. Some people think it inhibits spontaneity; however, I think you can incorporate it during foreplay. Your boyfriend can be the one who places it in the vagina.

Other forms of birth control that do not contain hormones include condoms, contraceptive gels (one that is prescribed and the others that you can buy in the store), and the cervical cap that works somewhat like the diaphragm. You can also consider permanent sterilization if you have decided to stop having children. For women who want permanent sterilization, we now remove the fallopian tubes completely. Studies have shown by removing the tubes, it may reduce the chances of developing ovarian cancer.

Rachel, I am not trying to tell you how many children you should have. It is none of my business. I just believed this would be the best time to discuss your options, since you are currently pregnant. Once the baby is born, it will be hard to think about your options, as you will be focused on the baby. I look forward to seeing you for your 28-week prenatal appointment. We will be checking your blood sugar levels during this visit, so be prepared to be in the office for at least one hour.

Sincerely,

Ngozi Osuagwu, MD, FACOG

NFertility awareness-based methods (FABMs) were most commonly referred to as natural family planning (NFP), which the World Health Organization defines as "methods for planning for avoiding pregnancies by observation of the natural signs and symptoms of fertile and infertile phases of the menstrual cycle."

To use FABMs to avoid pregnancy, you must not have sex during the fertile window.

For this method to work, you must have adequate instructions, be motivated, and have good cooperation and support from the male partner.

For the couple who wishes to have the slightest chance of pregnancy while using a FABM, it is prudent that intercourse is restricted to the postovulatory infertile phase, and two indicators are used to confirm the end of the fertile window. These indicators include checking the cervical fluid, basal body temperature, and calendar calculations based on cycle length and prior ovulation days.

Although many apps claim to help avoid or achieve pregnancy, a 2016 systematic review of apps marketed for avoiding pregnancy demonstrated that the majority are not concordant with evidence-based fertility awareness methods.

Source: Duane M, Stanford JB, Porucznik CA, Vigil P. Fertility Awareness-Based Methods for Women's Health and Family Planning. Front Med (Lausanne). 2022;9:858977. Published 2022 May 24. doi:10.3389/fmed.2022.858977 (Accessed June 21, 2022).

REPEAT TEEN PREGNANCY

Dear Dee Dee,

Let us really be honest with ourselves right now. You are fooling yourself to believe this man loves you. He has six children with God knows how many different women and he is not paying child support for any of them. How can he? He does not have a job. You say he loves you. That is crap! He loves the fact that he is living with you and does not have to pay rent. I would love to shake some sense into you, but this is as close as I could get. You are working two jobs just to support yourself and your two children; I do not believe this is fair to the children.

You wonder why you have not been able to get pregnant with this man. Well, when people tell me there are no modern-day miracles, I think about you and I know there are miracles. God is intervening. He is telling you that you do not need to be pregnant, especially with this man.

Anyway, forget about what I think. I was telling you the truth when I told you your government insurance card does not cover infertility work-ups. I cannot help you get pregnant because I will not get paid.

Dee Dee, if this man truly loves you, he would encourage you to go back to school. He would be trying to find a job. He would be trying to help you. Having another baby does not define love.

You have been my patient for the past 10 years. You had your first child at 15 and your second at 17. Even with those two children, you were able to finish high school and become a certified medical assistant. You are a hardworking woman and a wonderful mother. I know you have been single for many years, but I promise there is someone out there who is better than what you currently have. He will not even help you with your children because he says they are not his. If a man loves you, he should love you and your children.

I care about what happens to you. When you left the office the other day, I was speechless. I was numb. I know you can do so much better for yourself. In the meantime, I have sent a prescription for prenatal vitamins to your pharmacy. Since you are having unprotected sex, you should be on vitamins that have adequate folic acid to protect the spine of the baby in case you do become pregnant.

I am always here for you. If you need to talk, do not hesitate to call the office or schedule an appointment.

Sincerely,

Ngozi Osuagwu, MD, FACOG

One in five births to teen mothers aged 15–19 years is a repeat birth.

About 183 repeat teen births occur each day in the United States.

Infants born from a repeat teen birth are often born too small or too soon, which can lead to more health problems for the baby.

Having more than one child as a teen can limit the teen mother's ability to finish her education or get a job.

Source: Centers for Disease Control and Prevention. Preventing Repeat Teen Births. Vital Signs, April 2013. https://www.cdc.gov/vitalsigns/teenpregnancy/index.html (Accessed August 21, 2021).

PREGNANCY

Dear Ms. Dawson,

Congratulations on your pregnancy! Thank you for contacting my office to schedule your first appointment. I wanted to share my philosophy with you regarding pregnancy before you establish care with me to ensure that I am the right doctor for you. I hope this information solidifies your choice and I look forward to seeing you in two weeks to begin your obstetric care.

Pregnancy is a normal part of life. Without procreation, humanity would halt. Most women do not need an obstetrician and could do well without one. About 10 percent of women really do need an obstetrician because their pregnancy can result in loss of life or significant morbidity to mother and baby. Since it is difficult to know in what category you might find yourself, everyone should see an obstetrician or some qualified health attendant during pregnancy. There are people in remote parts of the world making and birthing babies without reading all the books or seeing an obstetrician, instead relying on those that have gone before them to help them through. I tell you this because it does not matter how many books you read on what you need to do to prepare for this wonderful journey, things can happen. I am here to help decrease the chances any of those things happening to you.

If you have not been eating healthy, this may be the time to start. Remember, you are eating for two now. That does not mean that you eat twice as much as you have been eating—you will need additional calories, but not twice as much. You can probably increase your calories by 25 percent. I do not believe in crazy types of cravings. You do not have to send your significant other on a wild goose chase for ice cream covered with chocolate, pecans, jelly, and chocolate chip morsels. Craving fruits, vegetables, and water are part of a healthy pregnancy outcome.

This is also not the time to start training for the marathon if you have been a couch potato or it takes heaven and earth to get you to work out. If you were already a highly active woman, pregnancy should not make you skip a beat. For women in between these two extremes, it is important to do something. Most women choose to walk for about 30 minutes a day, five days a week. You can work toward this goal. Exercise will not hurt your baby.

I do not like to be called constantly. Please try to use common sense. Take the following quiz:

1. You are exercising vigorously and you start having abdominal cramps. Do you continue to exercise, or do you stop?

2. You are having sex and you start to bleed; do you continue to have sex, or do you stop?

3. If you are eating a certain food and every time you eat this particular food, you get sick, do you continue to eat that food, or do you stop?

I think it is pretty obvious that in each case you should stop. I do not think that you need to call me to hear me say "stop." You are probably asking yourself when do you call the doctor. When you come for your initial visit, we will review all of this.

Let me tell you in advance that I cannot look at your belly or tell by the heart rate whether you are having a boy or a girl. My goal and prayer, which I hope is yours, is to have a healthy baby.

I hope what I have told you does not scare you. If you wish to keep your appointment, then I will see you in two weeks. If you are not interested in seeing me, I wish you well. Prenatal care is extremely important. Please schedule an appointment with your new provider as soon as possible and cancel your appointment with me so that another patient can be scheduled.

Sincerely,

Ngozi Osuagwu, MD, FACOG

The death of a woman during pregnancy, at delivery, or soon after delivery is a tragedy for her family and for society as a whole. Sadly, about 700 women die each year in the United States as a result of pregnancy or delivery complications.

The U.S. maternal mortality rate has more than doubled from 7.2 per 100, 000 live births in 1987 to 17.3 per 100,000 live births in 2017.

When combined, cardiovascular conditions (i.e., cardiomyopathy, other cardiovascular conditions, and cerebrovascular conditions) were responsible for more than one-third of pregnancy-related deaths in 2014–2017.

Black women are three times more likely to die in childbirth than are white women, regardless of education, income, or any other socioeconomic factors.

Source: Centers for Disease Control and Prevention. Reproductive Health: Pregnancy Mortality Surveillance System. https://www. cdc.gov/reproductivehealth/maternal-mortality/pregnancy-mortality-surveillance-system.htm#trends (Accessed August 21, 2021).

BREASTFEEDING

Dear Desiree,

You are 38 weeks pregnant, and I know each time we have discussed breastfeeding, you have been averse to it. You mentioned that you did not breastfeed your other child and that child turned out well. You also mentioned you were concerned about how your breasts would look after you had a baby suck on your nipples for even a day, let alone a year, and that your husband enjoys firm breasts and you did not want them sagging.

I obviously cannot force you to breastfeed, but I do want you to be aware of some of the benefits breastfeeding provides for you and your baby. For you, the best part is the weight loss. The weight which you gained during pregnancy generally comes off more quickly when you breastfeed. You can eat almost anything you want and not gain weight. Breast milk is free and comes in a wonderful package, so you do not have to worry about washing bottles. Additionally, some breastfeeding women do not have their periods, which can be a convenience. Regarding the shape of your breasts, that is all in the genes. There are women who have never had children and have sagging breasts, and there are people who have breastfed and feel that their breasts are firmer now than they were before.

For the baby, breast milk is a good source of antibodies that come from you to help prevent diseases. Breastfed babies generally get sick less and are less likely to die during the first year of life. They tend not to be overweight when they get older, and they are less prone to chronic illnesses like diabetes and asthma when they become adults. Breast milk is ever-changing, meeting the nutritional needs of the baby through every stage of development.

I know you are concerned because you did not breastfeed your first child and you do not want that child to feel they were not loved. I know you do not want to feel guilty. With every subsequent pregnancy, there will be options that were not available with the previous pregnancy. You are more knowledgeable now, and that counts. I think it would be worse to learn about the benefits of breastfeeding and not try it with this baby. It does not lessen the love you have for your first child.

Regarding your husband's likes and dislikes, let us not forget the real purpose of the breast. Like other organs in the body, it has a purpose: our ears are for listening, our lungs are for breathing, our legs for walking, our eyes for seeing, and our breasts are for breastfeeding.

The hospital where you will have the baby is a designated Baby Friendly® hospital. While you are at the hospital, they will encourage you to breastfeed. When the baby is delivered, the baby will be placed on your chest, which is called skin-to-skin contact. In addition, the baby will not leave your room. This will allow you to learn your baby's feeding cues, which means you will be able to tell when your baby is hungry. Everything in the hospital is designed to help with bonding and allow for breastfeeding. Do not be alarmed, and do not think everyone is ganging up against you. There will be formula available in the hospital at your request. We just believe breastfeeding is a good thing and can make a difference in the health of you and the baby.

If you have any questions or want to talk some more, please call the office. We have several resources to help support you. We have our local La Leche League and the WIC Peer Counselors. I look forward to seeing you next week.

Take care,

Ngozi Osuagwu, MD, FACOG

Infants who are breastfed have reduced risks of asthma, obesity, type 1 diabetes, ear and respiratory infections, and sudden infant death syndrome (SIDS). Breastfeeding can also help lower a mother's risk of hypertension, type 2 diabetes, and ovarian and breast cancer.

Highlights from the 2020 Breastfeeding Report Card:

+ *Among infants born in 2017, 4 out of 5 (84.1%) started out breastfeeding. This high percentage of babies who start out breastfeeding shows that most mothers want to breastfeed and are trying to do so.*

+ *About half (46.9) were exclusively breastfeeding at 3 months.*

+ *Only one-third (35.3%) of infants were breastfeeding at 12 months.*

+ *Almost half (51%) of employers provide worksite lactation support programs.*

+ *Comprehensive hospital practices and policies that support breastfeeding have been shown to reduce medically unnecessary formula supplementation, reduce disparities in breastfeeding, and help give infants the best start in life*

Source: Centers for Disease Control and Prevention. *Breastfeeding Report Card – United States, 2020.* https://www.cdc.gov/breastfeeding/data/reportcard.htm (Accessed March 19, 2022).

TOBACCO USE AND PREGNANCY

Dear Lynette,

I have tried calling you, but the number we have on file has been disconnected. I am writing because my nurse informed me you were concerned about the antibiotics I prescribed—you were wondering whether they would hurt your baby. This is truly a legitimate concern. I am thrilled you are concerned about what may or may not hurt your baby.

The antibiotic I am prescribing is safe in pregnancy. It is being used to treat you for a urinary tract infection. Although you do not feel like you have a bladder infection, bladder infections during pregnancy can be very serious if left untreated. We do not have to wait for you to have symptoms before we treat for a bladder infection. Please take the antibiotics as prescribed. You should take it twice a day, one in the morning and one in the evening, for the full seven days.

While we are on the topic of safety, I would like to remind you that smoking cigarettes is not good for your baby. You are seven months pregnant and continue to smoke. Cigarettes contain several harmful ingredients that are found in materials that you should not have in your body—nicotine (insecticide), butane (lighter fluid), cadmium (batteries), stearic acid (candle wax), hexamine (barbecue lighter), toluene (industrial solvents), ammonia (toilet cleaner), methanol (fuel), arsenic (poison), methane (sewer gas), lead, and carbon monoxide, just to name a few.

Smoking cigarettes can cause your baby to be small. It can also cause your baby to be born prematurely (earlier than the due date), leading to many other problems. The worse thing is it can cause your baby to die while still inside you. If the baby is born alive, the baby can have problems with its lungs which may cause the baby to have breathing problems. The baby can also have difficulty learning. It also increases the likelihood that the child will eventually become a smoker.

I know we have been talking about you quitting smoking. This really is important. There are several helplines available to help you quit. If you cannot quit cold turkey, we can even prescribe medication. Really think about quitting. I look forward to seeing you at your next scheduled appointment.

Sincerely,

Ngozi Osuagwu, MD, FACOG

Smoking and Pregnancy: Statistics

✦ *In 2016, 7.2% of women who gave birth smoked cigarettes during pregnancy.*

✦ *Prevalence of smoking during pregnancy was highest for women aged 20–24 years (10.7%), followed by women aged 15–19 years (8.5%) and 25–29 years (8.2%).*

✦ *Non-Hispanic American Indian or Alaska Native women had the highest prevalence of smoking during pregnancy (16.7%); non-Hispanic Asian women had the lowest (0.6%).*

✦ *The prevalence of smoking during pregnancy was highest among women with a completed high school education (12.2%) and second highest among women with less than a high school education (11.7%).*

✦ *Maternal tobacco use during pregnancy has been linked to a host of negative infant and child outcomes, including low birthweight, preterm birth, and various birth defects.*

Source: Centers for Disease Control and Prevention, National Center for Health Statistics. Cigarette Smoking During Pregnancy: United States, 2016. NCHS Data Brief No. 305, February 2018. https://www.cdc.gov/nchs/products/databriefs/db305.htm (Accessed August 21, 2021).

HUSBAND MATERIAL

Dear Nadesh,

I know you might read this letter and think to yourself, "what business does my physician have in my affairs?" but I will take my chances. I write because I have known you since you were a teenager and I care about you. You are now 28 years old, and I was bothered by your comment about your current boyfriend. You mentioned that he was not "husband material." I guess that would not have bothered me as much if you were using your birth control consistently. I just wonder how a man who is not "husband material" could be father material—or does it really matter? Fifty percent of pregnancies in the United States are unintended: they occur because people are not using birth control or are not using their birth control correctly. You are not taking your birth control pills daily. It is bound to fail one day, and if you are not ready to have a baby, then something needs to be done.

I know when we talked in the past, you have mentioned that one day, you would like to get married and have children. You have been dating your current boyfriend for two years. If you are interested in getting married one day, should you not be dating someone who is husband material? You moved in with this guy about six months ago to help with the rent. Cohabitating with him will truly limit your prospects. Men typically are not looking at women who are living with another man. Although they will date a woman whom they know has dated other men, by living with a man it is quite obvious you are in a relationship with him.

It is time to look at the big picture. You are 28 years old. Yes, you are young, but when do you think it will be time to start dating some-one who is "husband material"? It does not happen overnight. I have seen a lot of women think they have time, and by the time they are ready, it is too late. Suppose you get pregnant; this would also limit your prospects. I would hope the standard you have for a man to be a father is higher than the standard you have for him to be a boyfriend or husband, which would mean that you really must consider correctly using an effective birth control method. You also do not want to get into a situation where you get preg-nant and then you feel stuck— could you ever be happy?

That is it. I just needed to get it off my chest. No, I am not your mother, your older sister, nor your aunt. I am your physician and I care about you. Believe it or not, happiness plays such an import-ant role in one's health, and I want you to be happy. Please sched-ule an appointment to talk about a more effective birth control method that would not require much effort on your part. In the meantime, try using the alarm clock on your smartphone to re-mind you to take the birth control pills daily.

Sincerely,

Ngozi Osuagwu, MD, FACOG

LOOKING IN THE MIRROR

I looked in the mirror the other day and I saw this woman,

This beautiful woman,

And I wondered why I had never seen her before.

I wondered why it never occurred to me that she had a reason for living.

I wondered why it never occurred to me that she didn't need to have someone define her.

I wondered where she had been all this time.

Yes, I looked in the mirror the other day,

And oh my God,

I saw her.

I saw someone who needed to be here,

Someone who was meant to be.

MARRIED MAN

Dear Ms. Blake,

Why is it that some people need a hammer to hit them on the head before they believe that it is a hammer, while others are okay looking at a hammer and believing that it is a hammer, no demonstrations needed?

Ms. Blake, he is not leaving his wife for you. You have been dating him for three years, and each time you come to my office, you tell me it will happen soon, he is just waiting for the right time. After three years, do you not realize there is no right time?

To tell you the truth, I would not care if you came into the office and told me, "I am dating a married man and I love him, and I do not expect that he will divorce his wife." At least then I would say you are living in reality. But that is not the case; you have been waiting for three years, and by now it should be obvious he is not leaving his wife.

I want you to understand, every time you have sex with him you put yourself at risk for all types of diseases. You are at risk for any disease he has and any disease his wife might have, as well as those of any other person either of them sleeps with.

You have mentioned it is so hard to find a good man. You deserve better. You are a beautiful and talented young woman. I believe there is someone out there for you, but I believe it starts with you feeling good about yourself. You have to feel good about being with you and loving yourself. You will not be able to find the right person as long as you are infatuated with your current partner.

I know you probably did not expect a letter from your gynecologist discussing this issue, but you informed me during your office visit you have just been feeling stressed lately. When you were last seen in the office, your blood pressure was 138/90. It has never been that high. You have gained 20 pounds since your last visit, which was one year ago. I think your circumstance is contributing to the change in your health status. I do not want you to have higher blood pressure or be 20 pounds heavier at your next visit.

I have enclosed information on the DASH (dietary approaches to stopping hypertension) diet. It is designed to help with blood pressure and weight control. I would like you to follow this diet and to schedule a nurse visit in about three months for us to recheck your blood pressure and your weight. If you want to talk, I am here for you. Take care of yourself, and please consider what I have said.

Sincerely,

Ngozi Osuagwu, MD, FACOG

THE DASH DIET

DASH is a flexible and balanced eating plan that helps create a heart-healthy eating style for life.

The DASH eating plan requires no special foods and instead provides daily and weekly nutritional goals. This plan recommends:

✦ *Eating vegetables, fruits, and whole grains*

✦ *Including fat-free or low-fat dairy products, fish, poultry, beans, nuts, and vegetable oils*

✦ *Limiting foods that are high in saturated fat, such as fatty meats, full-fat dairy products, and tropical oils such as coconut, palm kernel, and palm oils*

✦ *Limiting sugar-sweetened beverages and sweets*

✦ *Limit the amount of sodium (salt)*

Source: National Institutes of Health, National Heart, Lung, and Blood Institute. DASH Eating Plan. https://www.nhlbi.nih.gov/health-topics/dash-eating-plan (Accessed August 18, 2021).

POLYCYSTIC OVARY SYNDROME (PCOS)

Dear Ms. Kagiso,

You came to me for a second opinion because you did not want to be labeled with a diagnosis. You had never heard of polycystic ovary syndrome. You had moved here about two years ago and prior to this you had been seeing a gynecologist for five years and they never said anything. The first gynecologist you saw when you moved here made the diagnosis and you were rather upset. I finally reviewed your lab work and based on the history I obtained from you and the physical exam at your last visit, I agree with your new gynecologist—you have polycystic ovary syndrome. The short name for this is PCOS.

I know this may come as a surprise, and you might be wondering why your other gynecologist never said anything. It can take years and sometimes requires seeing multiple gynecologists before the diagnosis is made.

The diagnosis of PCOS is usually one of exclusion, meaning we have to rule out all other possible reasons for your current symptoms. Typically the symptoms include irregular menstrual cycle, or for some women no menstrual cycle, abnormal hair growth, and at least one polycystic ovary (one with multiple small cysts inside) confirmed by ultrasound. You need at least two of these symptoms to be diagnosed with PCOS and we have to make sure nothing else can explain these symptoms.

I recall you also mentioned that you were not "fat" and according to your research, people with PCOS tend to be overweight. All women have the possibility of being diagnosed with PCOS regardless of their weight. Although majority of women who have PCOS tend to be overweight or obese, thin people can have PCOS.

Based on your history and physical exam, you actually have all three symptoms. You mentioned your periods have been irregular for the past five years, and although you liked not having a period every month, you cannot predict when you will have one so you always have to carry a pad. You also told me you have had an increase in facial hair that is requiring you to shave most mornings. You did not worry about that because all the women in your family are hairy. Lastly, the ultrasound revealed one of your ovaries is polycystic. It has what we call in the medical field "a ring of pearls." This is when we see follicles (little small cysts) around the ovary on the ultrasound image.

My recommendation is that you return to your gynecologist and discuss further management. I do not want you to go more than three months without a period, because that will put you at risk for precancer or cancer of the lining of the uterus. You will need to be screened for diabetes and high cholesterol. People with PCOS are at increased risk of chronic diseases in the future, and we want to detect things early. Finally, although it is true you are not obese, based on your body mass index, you are overweight and would benefit from exercising and being mindful of your diet.

Although PCOS increases your risk of developing certain serious health conditions, PCOS is not a death sentence. It is a chronic disease and can be managed. And yes, you will be able to have children; you just might require medication to help with ovulation. You will need to work with your gynecologist.

I hope I have explained everything in a way that is helpful to you. If you have any further questions for me, please do not hesitate to schedule an appointment.

Take care and all the best,

Ngozi Osuagwu, MD, FACOG

The incidence of PCOS varies according to the diagnostic criteria used.[1]

Using the National Institutes of Health Criteria, the incidence of PCOS is approximately 7% of reproductive-aged women.[1]

Obesity is not a diagnostic criterion for PCOS, and approximately 20% of women with PCOS are not obese.[1]

Polycystic ovaries appear to be inherited as an autosomal dominant trait: Among women who have PCOS, 3% to 35% of their mothers have PCOS.[2]

Sources: [1]*American College of Obstetricians and Gynecologists. Polycystic ovary syndrome. ACOG Practice Bulletin No. 194. Obstet Gynecol 2018;131:e157–e171;*

[2]*Rosenfield RL. The Diagnosis of Polycystic Ovary Syndrome in Adolescents. Pediatrics 2015;136:1154–1165.*

ENDOMETRIOSIS

Dear Ms. Alvarez,

I had a chance to review your records and understand why you are upset. It looks like you have been complaining of pain for the past three years and no one has been able to give you any answers. You have seen a urologist to check your bladder and a gastroenterologist to check your bowels, and they believe that your problem has to do with your pelvic organs. The last gynecologist wanted you to try birth control pills, but you were reluctant to take any medication without knowing your diagnosis.

As I mentioned to you in the office and now after reviewing your records, I suspect you have endometriosis. Endometriosis is where the type of cells that line the inside of your uterus is found outside of the uterus. You told me that over the past three years, your menstrual cycle is shorter and has become heavier. You also stated you have severe pain associated with your period and that ibuprofen no longer provides relief. You also said you continue to have pain beyond the time of your period, but it is not severe, and that you have pain with intercourse. You indicated you had an ultrasound that showed a cyst, but you do not recall the details and I did not see an ultrasound report in your records.

During your examination, you had some tenderness when I pressed down on your belly. When I performed your pelvic exam, I told you your uterus was tilted backward. It is what we call a retroverted uterus. The concern I had was that I really could not move your uterus freely and you had some tenderness. Your ovaries did not feel enlarged on my exam. Based on the exam, my diagnosis is leaning toward endometriosis.

Endometriosis is a chronic disease. The only way to make a definitive diagnosis is to take you to the operating room. We would perform a laparoscopy where we would make small incisions on your abdomen and put an instrument to look inside. Ideally, we would not only look inside to make the diagnosis, but we would remove as much endometriosis that is seen. Afterwards, you will need to be placed on medication. The goal of placing you on medication would be to prevent the symptoms you have been having, to prevent the endometriosis implants from coming back, and to minimize the need to perform multiple surgeries.

Another option is for me to try you on hormone medication and see how you do. I know it will not give you the definitive diagnosis that you want, but if you feel better, does it really matter? I can start you on a birth control pill, the shot, the implant, or the hormonal intrauterine device and see how it works. There is also a medication that came out particularly for endometriosis. I am comfortable prescribing this medication without taking you to surgery because your symptoms sound so convincing for endometriosis.

I know you have seen many physicians and have become frustrated. I want to work with you. Before anything else is done, I would like you to get a pelvic ultrasound to see if you still have the cyst you mentioned. Afterward, you will need to decide what you want to do next. If you decide to have surgery, I will refer you to a specialist. The reason I will not do the surgery is that I do not want a situation in which I look inside and the endometriosis is too extensive for me to burn away the disease and I close you back up without being able to remove the endometriosis. I believe if you are taken to surgery knowing there is a high probability of finding endometriosis, then we should plan for surgical removal of the endometriosis. Your endometriosis might be so extensive that removal would be better than just burning it away. After the surgery, I would start you on medical therapy immediately.

Please consider your options and let me know what you decide. I look forward to hearing from you soon. Take care.

Sincerely,

Ngozi Osuagwu, MD, FACOG

Endometriosis affects 6–10% of reproductive-aged women and has been found in both premenarchal and postmenopausal women.

The average age of diagnosis is approximately 28 years.

Endometriosis is present in 71–87% of those with chronic pelvic pain.

> *Source: Falcone T, Flyckt R. Clinical Management of Endometriosis. Obstet Gynecol 2018;1313:557–571.*

MULTIPLE SCLEROSIS

Dear Ms. Davidson,

I just received the letter from the neurologist informing me you have been diagnosed with multiple sclerosis (MS). The neurologist mentioned you were devastated and felt I should reach out to you sooner rather than later. She mentioned that you were concerned because your wedding was in two months and you were not sure you wanted to go through with it. She knows you have been my patient for twelve years and you are more of a friend than a patient, so it might be easier for me to communicate with you.

First let me tell you, I already bought a dress for the wedding and have no plans of returning it. You will get married in two months. There have been so many strides in treatment made when it comes to multiple sclerosis. I know what frightens you is the grandmother of one of your students who has MS and is wheelchair bound, but that does not have to be your fate. People can live wonderful and productive lives with MS. And yes, you will be able to start that family you have always wanted.

I am so happy you saw the neurologist. You mentioned your symptoms did not make sense to you. When your leg gave out a few months ago you believed you probably slipped on something and didn't think anything of it. Then you had a couple of episodes where you had blurred vision and thought you were probably due for an eye examination. I think what finally did it for you, is when you had weird tremors and one of your colleagues asked if you were using some type of drugs. Now you have seen the neurologist and have a diagnosis, these symptoms make sense, and you can focus on the plan for managing your type of MS.

There are four types of MS: relapsing-remitting, secondary progressive, primary progressive, and the clinically isolated syndrome. The neurologist believes that you have relapsing-remitting MS, which is the most common type. With relapsing-remitting MS, you typically have attacks over some days or weeks and then your symptoms completely go away for a time. The neurologist wants to start you on medication, which I believe is a great idea. She knows you do not plan on becoming pregnant for another two years and states she will place you on a medication that will not be a problem even if you want to become pregnant earlier than planned.

I urge you to consider bringing your fiancé to your next appointment with the neurologist. He probably has questions, and when you are in a relationship, although you are the one with the diagnosis of MS, it will affect both of you. The most important thing you can do is always keep the line of communication open with your doctors and with your life partner.

Please call me if there is anything I can do for you. Since your hormone-releasing intrauterine device is safe to use in women with MS, you do not need to remove it, and I do not need to see you in the office until next year unless anything changes. I will, however, see you at the wedding.

Take care.

Sincerely,

Ngozi Osuagwu, MD, FACOG

Multiple sclerosis (MS) can occur at any age from childhood to 80 years, but the average age of onset is 34 years.

Approximately 400,000 individuals in the United States and nearly 2.3 million individuals worldwide have MS.

The disease affects three times as many females as males.

The causes of MS remain unknown.

Source: Fang X, Patel C, Gudesblatt M. Multiple Sclerosis: Clinical Updates in Women's Health Care Primary and Preventive Care Review. Obstet Gynecol 2020;135:757–758.

DIABETES AND YEAST INFECTION

Dear Ms. Thomas,

You mentioned in the office you were scared to start on insulin because most of your relatives who started on insulin therapy ended up having their legs amputated. Ms. Thomas, it is not the insulin that caused the amputation, it is the fact their blood sugar was not controlled.

Today was the third time this year you have come to me with complaints of severe itching. The cause of your itching is a yeast infection. You will continue to have yeast infections that cause symptoms as long as your sugars are not controlled. Although you told me you have been checking your sugars and they have been good, I checked your hemoglobin A1c and it was high. It was 10.2. Ideally, you want your hemoglobin A1c to be less than 6.5. The hemoglobin A1c tells me how well your blood sugar has been controlled over the past three months. The only reason I checked was because you kept telling me I was not treating you properly and that is why you keep getting yeast infections.

As long as your blood sugar is high, you will continue to have yeast infections. I will definitely get a prescription to your pharmacy for the fluconazole; you should take one when you get your prescription filled and the other tablet in 72 hours. I would also like you to schedule an appointment to see your primary care physician. Just because you begin taking insulin now does not mean that you will need insulin for the rest of your life. You just need some additional help right now. I also think it is time you see a dietician to go over your diet.

You might not realize it, but some of the community centers nearby have a diabetic program that includes education on how to manage diabetes. Some of these programs are free or low cost depending on your income. I think it is time you take advantage of these programs.

If I can be of further assistance, please do not hesitate to contact the office. I look forward to seeing you in a couple of months for your annual well woman exam.

Sincerely,

Ngozi Osuagwu, MD, FACOG

Diabetes Statistics[1]

Approximately one out of every ten people in the United States has diabetes.

One out of five people with diabetes is not aware of their condition.

People who have diabetes are at a higher risk of serious health complications such as blindness, kidney failure, heart disease, stroke, and loss of toes, feet, or legs.

One out of three adults has prediabetes.

Eight out of ten people with prediabetes do not know they have it.

If you have prediabetes, losing weight by eating healthy and being more active can reduce your risk of getting diabetes by 50%.

National Diabetes Prevention Program[2]

The National Diabetes Prevention Program (DPP) is a public–private partnership offering evidence-based, low-cost interventions in communities across the United States to prevent type 2 diabetes. The year-long program provides participants with a trained lifestyle coach, CDC-approved curriculum, and group support designed to help them make beneficial lifestyle changes.

Sources: [1]Centers for Disease Control and Prevention. A Snapshot: Diabetes in the United States. https://www.cdc.gov/diabetes/library/socialmedia/infographics/diabetes.html (Accessed August 18, 2021);

[2]Centers for Disease Control and Prevention. What is the National DPP? https://www.cdc.gov/diabetes/prevention/about/index.html (Accessed August 18, 2021).

VULVA CARE

Dear Ms. Hastings,

I do not know what to say anymore. If you are not willing to listen to my advice, there is not much more I can offer you. For the past six months, you have been coming to me because of irritation on your vulva. You mentioned your other doctor had treated you for bacterial vaginosis and yeast infections in the past and your symptoms seemed to get better but then the infection would come back again. You do not have any of the three common causes of vaginitis. You do not have a yeast infection, you do not have bacterial vaginosis, and you do not have trichomoniasis. Ms. Hastings, you have some type of contact dermatitis. I believe you are allergic to something; I am just not sure what it is. You must be willing to follow my advice. I just need you to follow my advice for at least one month so we can see what is happening.

When it comes to the vulva—I know you like to call it "down there"—you need to keep it simple. Please make sure you are wearing cotton underwear. In the past you told me the crotch was cotton—you need the whole undergarment to be cotton. Pack away the thongs. Pack away the silky underwear. You have got to trust me on this one. The next thing I need you to do is change your soap. I know you love the fragranced soaps, but you are going to need to let those go at least for now. I prefer you use an unscented soap that has some moisturizing cream.

The next thing you have to do is to stop douching. I know you mentioned you stopped douching after your period years ago, but you felt you needed to so after intercourse. As I have told you during several previous visits, if you cannot stand the ejaculate that comes from your partner, maybe you should not be having sex with that partner. You may even consider using a condom. There is absolutely no reason to douche after your partner ejaculates. You have to let that go.

The other big one for you is hair removal. Hair really does have a purpose, and you seem to want to get a Brazilian more often than recommended. Please stop waxing. You might find this one thing stops the irritation you are having.

Remember, I am asking you to do all of this for a month. After the month, I will reassess how you are feeling. You really need to give it a try and do everything I have communicated to you before you say it does not work. Keep a diary of how you feel each day. If you have any questions, please do not hesitate to contact me.

Sincerely,

Ngozi Osuagwu, MD, FACOG

Vulva Care Guidelines

✦ Use unscented laundry detergent.

✦ Do not use fabric softeners or dryer sheets.

✦ Use hypoallergenic/unscented body bar soap.

✦ Wear cotton underwear (no thongs, preferably white underwear).

✦ Do not use dry weave menstrual pads.

✦ DO NOT douche.

✦ Limit shaving of the vulva area (limit to bikini line only).

"LIVING IN YOUR VAGINA"

Dear Ms. Nelson,

An apology is probably warranted for the comment I made. When I said you needed to "stop living in your vagina," it just came out, and I should not have said that. I do not want to discourage you from being in tune with your body. I made the comment in frustration and I apologize.

I have seen you seven times in the past six months. The first time you had vaginal itching with a white cottage cheese–like discharge. I looked at it under the microscope. You definitely had a yeast infection. I explained to you it was not sexually transmitted and that your partner did not need to be treated. During the visit, I tested you for gonorrhea, chlamydia, and trichomoniasis and the results were negative. I did not perform a Pap smear because you were not due to have one. You left that boyfriend and met another guy one month later. You came to me because you noted an odor with your discharge, and you mentioned you were spotting. You swore when you told me you were using condoms. This time I diagnosed you with trichomoniasis. This is sexually transmitted, and I gave you antibiotics and told you your partner needed to be treated. I once again checked you for gonorrhea and chlamydia and both tests were negative. You left this man and met another guy. The next three times you came in because you were nervous and wanted to make sure you did not have another sexually transmitted infection. You did not trust your current boyfriend. You thought you might have had a discharge, but you were not sure, and you just wanted to make sure you did not have anything.

I am not sure I understand why you would be in a relationship with someone you do not trust? You have been in my office almost every month since you have been with him. You check your underwear all the time. You are scared you might itch, but you are not itching. I do not think it is worth it to be in this relationship.

I am not saying that I will not see you. But I will not treat you for something you do not have. You have discharge, but all women have physiologic discharge. Your discharge also changes depending on your cycle. You will notice a thin discharge immediately after your period, and then about mid-cycle, the discharge becomes very thick and stringy. It still remains clear. It then becomes a little less thick as we get closer to our period.. These changes are based on hormonal changes during your cycle. This is normal. Just like some women are short and some women are tall, some women have more of this physiologic discharge than others.

It is not normal to have odor, and it is not normal to have itching associated with your discharge. It is not normal to have a foul-smelling period or menstrual flow. In your case, you do not have anything but worry. Yes, you had a yeast infection earlier, and yes, you had trichomoniasis earlier, but you have nothing now. I have tested you for gonorrhea, chlamydia, and trichomoniasis at least six times, and the results have been negative. I have performed a wet mount at least six times, and you do not have bacterial vaginosis or a yeast infection. I have also checked you for herpes, and your blood test came back negative.

Ms. Nelson, your options include leaving your current partner and moving on or continuing to do what you have been doing (which in essence is "living in your vagina"). If you do not believe what I am telling you, you can seek a second opinion and that is quite okay.

I know that you have been reluctant to use condoms because you have mentioned that you are allergic to latex and the plastic condoms are much more expensive and just do not feel the same. I know you are on a reliable form of birth control, the implant, so you have not needed to use condoms for contraception, but I really believe using condoms may help relieve some of your anxiety.

Again, please do not get offended. You are a wonderful patient and I want to continue to be your doctor. If you have any questions regarding this letter, please feel free to schedule another appointment so we can discuss it.

Sincerely,

Ngozi Osuagwu, MD, FACOG

Facts About Vaginitis

+ *Vaginitis is defined as inflammation or infection of the vagina and is associated with a spectrum of symptoms, including vulvovaginal itching, burning, irritation, dyspareunia (painful sex), "fishy" vaginal odor, and abnormal vaginal discharge.*

+ *The most common causes of vaginitis are bacterial vaginosis (22–50% of women with symptoms); vulvovaginal candidiasis, or yeast infection (17–39% of women with symptoms); and trichomoniasis (4–35% of women with symptoms).*

+ *Other causes of vaginitis symptoms include vulvar skin diseases, desquamative inflammatory vaginitis, and genitourinary syndrome of menopause.*

+ *Vaginitis may remain undiagnosed in 7 – 72% of patients.*

+ *In order to be treated successfully, an accurate diagnosis is required.*

Source: Vaginitis in Nonpregnant Patients: ACOG Practice Bulletin, Number 215. Obstet Gynecol. 2020 Jan;135(1):e1-e17. doi: 10.1097/AOG.0000000000003604. PMID: 31856123.
https://www.acog.org/clinical/clinical-guidance/practice-bulletin/articles/2020/01/vaginitis-in-nonpregnant-patients
(Accessed August 18, 2021)

INFERTILITY

Dear Ms. N'Diaye,

When you left the office, I could sense that you were down. I do not feel you were listening to what I was saying, so I thought I would send you this letter. First, you should not regret waiting until now to start having a child. I know you and your husband dated for six years before getting married, and then both of you decided to wait for another year before trying to have a baby. I know you expected to get pregnant immediately, like most of your friends, once you stopped the pills. Everyone is so different. I know you and your husband have been trying for the past eight months as I have continued the infertility evaluation, but it is time for your husband to submit a semen analysis.

You keep beating yourself up, thinking the reason you are not able to have a child is your fault. Let me remind you, male factor is a cause of infertility in 40- 50 % of couples. It does not matter your husband fathered a child when he was a teenager. He fathered the child over 20 years ago, and a lot can change in 20 years. Also, in the end, we can do all the workup and not have a cause of why you have been unable to conceive. Of couples experiencing infertility, up to 30% are unexplained which means we do not have a cause for their infertility.

Here is where we stand with your workup. Your menstrual cycle is about every 28 – 32 days. I have checked your progesterone level during the latter part of your cycle to confirm you are ovulating, and the progesterone level shows that you are ovulating. I know it may seem obvious, and I am not trying to insult you, but the only time you can get pregnant is by having sex around the time you are ovulating. You and your husband live busy lives, and he is always traveling. If you are not having sex at that critical time, you will not get pregnant.

You have been talking a lot about your aging ovaries. Your ovaries are not menopausal. I checked the follicular stimulating hormone (FSH) and the antimullerian hormone (AMH) levels, and your ovaries are functioning well.

We have known about your uterine fibroids since your late 20s. They have not grown. The ultrasound that was performed showed you have two fibroids located within the walls of the uterus, and they have been the same size for years. The hysterosalpingogram (HSG) test showed dye going through both tubes, which indicated the tubes were patent (open). It also showed no fibroids within the cavity of the uterus. Usually, the fibroids within the uterine cavity may cause problems with fertility. Many women with uterine fibroids have gotten pregnant without having surgery to remove fibroids. Taking you for surgery to remove those two fibroids would not make a difference based on the findings.

Your uterus, ovaries, and tubes are ready for you to become pregnant. Once your husband submits his semen analysis, I can discuss the next steps. I suspect that we may end up not finding a cause. If this is the case, I usually will end up sending you to an infertility specialist. These gynecologists have spent additional years of training in reproductive medicine. For unexplained infertility, you will need ovulating stimulating medication and intrauterine insemination (IUS). We do not perform IUS in our office. Once you become pregnant, the infertility specialist will send you back to me to take care of your pregnancy.

Please do not be discouraged. I am a prayerful woman and will keep you and your husband in my prayers. You have done nothing wrong but try to make sure that your little one 'to be' will come into a loving family. Please have your husband read the instructions provided to you at the visit and submit his semen analysis. Continue to take your prenatal vitamin. Once I get the results, we can set up an appointment to discuss the next steps.

Sincerely,

Ngozi Osuagwu, MD, FACOG

Infertility, defined as failure to achieve pregnancy within 12 months of unprotected intercourse or therapeutic donor insemination in women younger than 35 years or within 6 months in women older than 35 years, affects 15 % of couples.

Male factor is a cause of infertility in 40 – 50% of couples.

Unexplained infertility maybe diagnosed in as many as 30 % of infertile couples.

Source: Infertility Workup for the Women's Health Specialist: ACOG Committee Opinion, Number 781. Obstet Gynecol. 2019;133(6):e377-e384. doi:10.1097/AOG.0000000000003271 (Accessed May 23, 2022)

SEXUAL PROBLEMS

Dear Ms. Roberts,

I know that when you left the office yesterday after your annual exam, you were upset and that is why I am writing today. When you scheduled your appointment, you scheduled it as an annual exam. When I came into the room, I asked whether you had any concerns and you said no. When I was updating your chart, I specifically asked about your husband and whether you had any concerns regarding sex. After the physical exam, I focused on your weight because I noticed you had gained 15 pounds since your last visit. You mentioned since you became menopausal, it had become difficult to maintain your weight. We spent some time discussing ways to maintain your weight so you would not be 15 pounds heavier at your next visit. After I had spent 30 minutes in the office and was ready to leave the room, you stopped me and said, "By the way doctor, sex has not been the same for the past year, but I was embarrassed to say anything."

First, you should never feel embarrassed to talk with your physician about anything, especially when your physician specifically inquired about your sexual relationship with your husband. Second, sexual problems are not problems that can be addressed in a five-minute session. It requires me to get a comprehensive history. I need to ask more questions. What does it mean when you say sex has not been the same for the past year? Do you have problems with desire? Is it a problem with arousal? Have you been able to have an orgasm? Are you having pain? Each problem is handled differently because the causes for each problem differ. Also, are you having problems with the relationship? Do you still like your husband? Have you fallen out of love?

Sex is a very important part of life. I do not think you ever get too old to have sex. The method may be different, but the need for closeness and companionship is important. I did not want to blow you off. I needed time to discuss the problem thoroughly.

Please schedule an appointment so that I can address your concerns about sex. I have listed the questions that I will need to ask. Be prepared to answer those questions when you come in. It might help to write your answers on a sheet of paper and have it ready for the office visit. We can then spend time addressing the problem and working on solutions.

Sincerely,

Ngozi Osuagwu, MD, FACOG

Sexual dysfunction is a problem that prevents you wanting and enjoying sexual activity.

Approximately 40% of women will experience some type of sexual problem over the course of their lifetime.

It can occur at any age, but most common in women over the age of 40 years old.

Sexual dysfunction can affect your quality of life.

Physicians will not always ask the question, so you must be willing to talk about the problem.

Source: Simon JA, et al. *Distressing Sexual Function at Midline: Unmet Needs, Practical Diagnoses, and Available Treatments.* Obstet Gynecol 2017;130(4):889–905.

PAP SMEAR WITH HUMAN PAPILLOMAVIRUS (HPV) TEST

Dear Nguyen,

I have tried calling you several times, but it seems as if we have been playing telephone tag. This is why I decided to write to you. My nurse told me you were concerned because you did not receive the results of your Pap smear and it had been at least two months since your visit.

I think you may have forgotten what we had discussed at your last visit. Although you came to the office for an annual exam and I performed a pelvic exam, I did not obtain a Pap smear. A Pap smear is a screening test for cervical cancer, and for the majority of women, it does not have to be obtained every year. In your case, you had a Pap smear and human papillomavirus (HPV) test which were negative about two years ago. You are not due for a Pap smear for another three years. Women over 30 years of age who have had a Pap smear with the HPV test and both are negative will get a Pap smear with HPV test every five years. I know it may seem scary to wait so long between tests, but we know so much more about cervical cancer than we did in the past. Nearly 100 percent of cervical cancers are caused by HPV. When the Pap smear and HPV tests are negative, your chance of having something abnormal within five years is very, very small. We no longer obtain Pap smears yearly unless you have had a history of precancerous cells or have had cervical cancer. We also perform yearly Pap smears on women whose immune system is not working very well; for example, women who are HIV positive or women taking medication to suppress their immune system because they have had an organ transplant. If you desire to have the pap smear earlier than five years, I can obtain a pap smear earlier, but not earlier than three years in your case.

What people often forget is the Pap smear is performed to find abnormalities in cervical cells before it turns into cancer. The Pap smear does not prevent precancerous cells. Performing a Pap smear every year will not prevent precancerous cells from occurring. We can prevent precancerous cells by changing our behavior. We can wait until we are older before having sex. We can get the HPV vaccine before we start having sex. We can limit the number of sexual partners we have. We can stop smoking. I know that you were concerned because your cousin had cervical cancer. Cervical cancer is not hereditary. Remember, you said that your cousin had not seen a gynecologist for 10 years prior to being diagnosed with cervical cancer. The Pap test is one of the best screening tests we have in medicine, but it can only help prevent cervical cancer if you get it; however, you do not need to get it every year.

My role as a gynecologist is not limited to performing only Pap smears. Remember that I am your only physician since you do not have a family doctor. Each year when you come in, I review all the changes that might have happened since your last yearly exam. If you are having problems with your period, we discuss how it can be managed. This is the time we discuss whether you are happy with your current form of birth control. I review your exercise routine and make sure that you are maintaining a healthy weight. I make sure that you are up to date with your vaccinations. You were due to have your tetanus shot with pertussis at your last visit, so we gave you the vaccine. I also make sure that you are staying up to date with your dentist and optometrist appointments.

I also performed a physical exam. This year, I noticed a lump in your left breast. I received a letter from the breast surgeon you saw and was informed the biopsy was benign (it did not show cancer).

You are 37 years old and have been doing well. You have done all the right things to decrease your risk factors for most diseases. I know we cannot prevent all diseases, but we can hopefully discover most diseases early to help prevent any of the complications that might occur due to the disease.

If you have any questions or concerns, please do not hesitate to contact the office. I look forward to seeing you next year.

Sincerely,

Ngozi Osuagwu, MD, FACOG

Cervical cancer is most frequently diagnosed in women between the ages of 35 and 44 with the average age at diagnosis being 50. It rarely develops in women younger than 20.[1]

More than 20% of cases of cervical cancer are found in women over 65.[1]

As many as 93% of cervical cancer cases could be prevented by screening (Pap smear and/or HPV testing) and HPV vaccination.[2]

Sources: [1]American Cancer Society. *Key Statistics for Cervical Cancer.* https://www.cancer.org/cancer/cervical-cancer/about/key-statistics.html (Accessed August 19, 2021); [2]Centers for Disease Control and Prevention. *Cervical Cancer is Preventable. Vital Signs,* November 2014. https://www.cdc.gov/vitalsigns/cervical-cancer/index.html (Accessed August 19, 2021).

HUMAN IMMUNODEFICIENCY VIRUS

Dear Ms. Lackey,

I wanted to inform you I have sent your records to the University. It is not that I have a problem taking care of you, but the University actually has an human immunodeficiency virus (HIV) clinic and has had wonderful results in terms of decreasing the risk of HIV transmission from you to your unborn child. They have a team that will work with you, and they have incredible resources. I believe it would be in your best interest to continue your prenatal care at the University. Once you have delivered, you can come back to this practice for your gynecologic care.

I also want to take this opportunity to apologize for any misunderstanding that you might have had regarding having the HIV test performed. I recall, in the past, you have always declined testing when I offered. You mentioned you had been with your husband exclusively for the past 10 years and prior to your wedding, both of you tested negative. You and your husband did not engage in drug use. You have used condoms every time you have engaged in vaginal intercourse except during the months that you were ready to start a family. You said that you occasionally had anal intercourse, only in the past two years, but that you often did not use condoms because you figured you could not get pregnant having anal sex.

We have a standard set of labs we order for new obstetrical patients. HIV testing is recommended for all pregnancies. I forgot to remove the HIV test at your request. Once again, I am sorry; however, in some ways this may have been a good thing. This is your first pregnancy, and as I mentioned in the office visit, we can essentially prevent the baby from becoming HIV positive with the interventions we have available.

HIV is a reportable condition where we live. By law, you are required to inform your husband of the results. I know this will be a difficult discussion and I am available to assist. It will be very important your husband gets tested.

Please call me if you have any questions. You will definitely be in good hands at the University for your obstetric care, and as I mentioned, if you wish, you may return to our practice for gynecologic care after you deliver.

Sincerely,

Ngozi Osuagwu, MD, FACOG

About 154,000 people (14%) who have HIV don't know it and need testing.[1]

About 37% of people who know they have HIV don't have it under control and need treatment.[1]

About 4 in 5 (82%) people who could benefit from medicine to prevent HIV (PrEP –Pre-exposure prophylaxis) aren't getting it.[1]

Advances in HIV research, prevention, and treatment have made it possible for many women with HIV to give birth to babies who are free of HIV. The annual number of HIV infections through perinatal transmission (mother to child) has declined by more than 95% since the early 1990s.[2]

The risk of transmitting HIV to your baby can be less than 1% or less if you take the following measures:[2]

✦ Take HIV medicine daily as prescribed throughout pregnancy, labor, and delivery.

✦ Give HIV medicine to your baby for 4–6 weeks after giving birth.

Sources: [1]Centers for Disease Control and Prevention. Ending HIV transmission. Test, Treat and Prevent. Vital Signs. Dec 2019. https://www.cdc.gov/vitalsigns/test-treat-prevent/index.html (Accessed August 19, 2021);

[2]Centers for Disease Control and Prevention. HIV and Pregnant Women, Infants, and Children. https://www.cdc.gov/hiv/group/gender/pregnantwomen/index.html (Accessed August 19, 2021).

UTERINE FIBROIDS (NEWLY DIAGNOSED)

Dear Ms. Davis

I am writing you as a follow-up to your visit. I received the ultrasound report and reviewed the images—you do have uterine fibroids. I know that you were worried. You mentioned you have been seeing doctors and none of them ever told you that you had fibroids. I cannot talk to you about what happened in the past; I can only tell you, when I saw you two weeks ago, as a new patient for an annual exam your uterus felt enlarged as if you were two months pregnant. You mentioned you have been on birth control pills for the past two years and the pills have helped with your menstrual cramps and bleeding.

Uterine fibroids are benign tumors, meaning they are growths within the uterus that are not cancerous. We do not completely understand why some women get them and others do not, but there is research being done. Black women tend to have a high risk of having fibroids, and it tends to happen to us when we are younger. Our symptoms also tend to be worse than those of other ethnic groups. Symptoms include heavy menstrual flow and severe cramps. You are on birth control pills, so this is probably helping with your symptoms. Some women can have very large fibroids where they look pregnant, and this can be associated with pelvic pressure causing them to urinate a lot or even have problems having bowel movements.

I know you mentioned that you were worried about having children in the future. Women with fibroids can have children. It is hard to predict what will happen, in your case, until you start trying to get pregnant. I know you were also worried about the fibroids growing; it is hard to predict what will happen. Fibroids can behave differently—some can have growth spurts, while others can shrink, and some can stay the same size. We know that when a woman reaches menopause, the fibroids should stop growing and some will even get smaller.

In the past, I would have told you there was nothing you should be doing now; however, the latest research suggests diet can play a role. A diet high in red meat is associated with growth of fibroids. Eating fruits and vegetables can be extremely helpful. Low-fat dairy products can be good. Also, making sure your vitamin D level is normal can be helpful. This was one of the reasons I drew blood from you. Your vitamin D level was low, so I have enclosed a prescription for a supplement.

I know you were also concerned about cancer. The cancer associated with fibroids is called leiomyosarcoma. This cancer usually occurs in older women, women on certain medications like Tamoxifen, and those women who have been exposed to pelvic irradiation. There might also be some genetic component, meaning it might run in families. This is not to say it does not happen to young people, but it is rare and having fibroids does not put you at increased risk compared with a woman who does not have fibroids. All women are at some risk.

I hope I have answered most of your questions. I really would encourage you to sign up with our electronic patient portal. It will allow you to have access to your results and to communicate with me more easily. I would like to see you in three months for a follow-up exam.

Sincerely,

Ngozi Osuagwu, MD, FACOG

Uterine fibroids (leiomyomas) are the most common tumors in women. By age 50, nearly 70% of white women and more than 80% of black women will have at least one fibroid.[1]

The decision regarding how to manage your uterine fibroids is a personal one and should be made with the knowledge and understanding of all available options.

Source: [1]Stewart EA. Uterine Fibroids. N Engl J Med 2015;372(17):1646–1655.

UTERINE FIBROIDS: FOURTH OPINION

Dear Ms. Okeke,

I am writing because you have an appointment to see me in two weeks for a fourth opinion. Typically, I wait until the day of your appointment to review the records, but because you were asking for a fourth opinion, I became curious. After reviewing the records, I agree with what your previous physicians recommended. I do not want you to waste your time or money coming to see me.

On review of your records, you are 52 years old and noticed about three years ago that your periods were heavier than usual. You were aware you had uterine fibroids for the past 10 years and actually had a myomectomy about seven years ago. You were doing well until recently, when the bleeding and the menstrual cramps became worse. You have four children and have no intention of having any more. Your first doctor suggested that you have a hysterectomy or take medication that would shrink the fibroids and possibly aid in making you go through menopause faster. You mentioned you were not interested in putting hormones in your body and wanted to have a myomectomy. He said that he would not perform a myomectomy, as you are not interested in having children and there is no need to preserve your uterus. He wanted you to seek a second opinion. The second opinion also felt you needed a hysterectomy and even suggested having your ovaries removed because of your age. Based on the notes, it appears that you were definitely not pleased with the second doctor's bedside manner and thought it was best to seek a third opinion. The third doctor was willing to perform a myomectomy but told you there was the possibility of having to do a hysterectomy—removal of the whole uterus—and you wanted to avoid that possibility.

I have found in my career when a patient has reached the point of seeking a fourth opinion, they are trying to find a doctor who will tell them what they want to hear. At your age, I do not believe there would be any benefit to having a myomectomy. I agree with your first doctor—your options include a hysterectomy and/or the medication that would help shrink your fibroids. I do not believe you need your ovaries removed; however, if you have a family history of breast or ovarian cancer, you may need to consider removing them. Also, if during the surgery the ovaries look suspicious, we would remove them. It is not unreasonable for the third physician to inform you that you may need a hysterectomy. You had a previous myomectomy and there is a chance you have scar tissue. This will make the surgery difficult. Also, with a myomectomy, you have a greater chance of bleeding than with a hysterectomy. It is not unreasonable to say that you might be at an increased risk of needing a hysterectomy.

There are other options, which I am not sure have been explored, such as uterine artery embolization, MRI (magnetic resonance imaging)—guided focused ultrasound surgery, and radiofrequency ablation. I could not sense from the records that these options were discussed with you. The first two of these options would be done by an interventional radiologist and the other I do not perform.

I probably could have waited for you to come into the office, but I thought it would be best to be honest with you. I do not want you to waste your time or money. In your case, I believe a hysterectomy is a good option. If you still want to talk or you want to establish care with me, please feel free to keep the appointment. If you choose not to come to the appointment, we would appreciate at least a 48- to 72-hours notice so that we can schedule another patient in that appointment slot.

Sincerely,

Ngozi Osuagwu, MD, FACOG

Getting My Hysterectomy

I do not need my uterus to make me feel like I'm a woman.

Who needs to bleed monthly and worry about accidents?

I was not so lucky to get it every 28 days, lasting for 3 days.

Mine decided to come every 21 days,

And run down like a waterfall

Lasting for 10 days and sometimes more.

And those damn cramps,

Did I tell you about them?

Keeping me bent over and helpless,

Unable to do anything worthwhile during that time.

Who needs that uterus to feel like a woman?

I know what makes me feel like a woman

It sure isn't this uterus.

I've made all my babies.

It has served its purpose.

And so I got the damn thing out.

No regrets.

I needed to enjoy the rest of my life.

Took the tubes out too,

No need for them.

Kept my ovaries,

I needed those hormones.

But I didn't need this uterus

To make me feel like I'm a woman.

BREAST CANCER

Dear Ms. Croft,

By the time you read this letter, you will have the biopsy results that reveal you have breast cancer. I have tried reaching you by telephone but have not been able to get through; therefore, I am writing to tell you that if you need anything, I am here. I also want to tell you that you did everything right.

I have known you for the past 10 years and you have been diligent about coming in for your exams every year. You have also been good about getting your mammogram yearly. I am so glad you called the office as soon as you felt the lump. You did not say to yourself, "Well, I just saw the doctor three months ago and everything was okay, so this must be nothing," or "I had a mammogram four months ago and it was normal." You called the office immediately and told us that you felt a lump on your left breast. We ordered a diagnostic mammogram and a left breast ultrasound the next day. You were immediately sent to a breast specialist based on the findings, and then you had the biopsy. Everything was done within a week of your telephone call.

You are 55 years old with three children and a grandchild on the way. I know you have been happily married for 25 years. I know you have never smoked or used any street drugs and you are a church-going, God-fearing woman. I know you do not have any family history of breast cancer. I know during the past two years, you have started to exercise and have been mindful of what you eat. I know the most logical question in your mind is, "Why me?" I wish I had the answer. I wish, as your doctor, I could wish the cancer away.

It is times like this I remember Psalm 121:1–2 NIV: "I lift up my eyes to the mountains – where does my help come from? My help comes from the Lord, the maker of heaven and earth." Ms. Croft, if you have any questions or just need someone to talk with, I am available. Please do not hesitate to call my office for any reason. Take care of yourself.

Sincerely,

Ngozi Osuagwu, MD, FACOG

About one in eight U.S. women (about 13%) will develop invasive breast cancer over the course of their lifetime.

About 85% of breast cancers occur in women who have no family history of breast cancer.

The most significant risk factors for breast cancer are gender (being a woman) and age (growing older).

For women in the United States, breast cancer death rates are higher than those for any other cancer other than lung cancer.

Breast cancer is the most commonly diagnosed cancer among American women.

In women younger 45 years, breast cancer is more common in Black women than white women. Overall, Black women are more likely to die of breast cancer. The risk of developing and dying from breast cancer is lower for Asian, Hispanic, and Native American women.

Source: Breastcancer.org. U.S. Breast Cancer Statistics. https://www.breastcancer.org/symptoms/understand_bc/statistics (Accessed August 19, 2021).

COLON CANCER SCREENING

Dear Ms. Falade,

It was a pleasure seeing you the other day. You are truly doing well. Your mammogram came back negative. I would recommend you get your mammogram yearly. Your pap smear and human papillomavirus (HPV) test were negative. Your next pap smear will be due in five years. This does not mean you do not see me for five years. You still need to see me for your general well woman exam annually.

My primary concern is you have not been screened for colon cancer. You are 53 years old, and for the past three years, I have been urging you to get screened for colon cancer. Colon cancer screening is very important. Colorectal cancer is the third leading cause of cancer death in women after lung and breast cancer. Colon cancer screening saves lives. We can find a problem in your colon before it becomes cancerous. The age for screening for colon cancer has changed from age 50 to now age 45. You are past due.

Although there are many options for screening, I prefer a colonoscopy. The reason is because if something is found, a biopsy can immediately be performed. I also like this test because it screens for the whole colon and not just part of the colon. Most people of color tend to get cancer on the right side of their colon, which is not easily detected with some other forms of screening.

I know you mentioned you had an aunt who had a complication

after having a colonoscopy. There is no doubt there are risks to having a colonoscopy. The risks include bleeding and perforation (making a hole in the colon. These risks are rare. When the colonoscopy is performed, it is extremely important your bowels are completely cleared of all stool and you go to an experienced physician. I can place the referral to the physician who performed my colonoscopy.

I have had a colonoscopy. The worst part of the procedure is the bowel prep before the procedure. I would recommend you schedule your colonoscopy on a Monday or Friday. You will need the day before to prep your bowels. You cannot do this at work. Believe me, I thought I could, and then I had to cancel my afternoon patients. Scheduling your procedure on a Monday or Friday minimizes the time off work. Also, try to get your procedure scheduled in the morning. You will need to have someone with you since you will be given medication that will make you sleepy, and you will not be able to drive. If your colonoscopy is completely normal, you may not need another one for ten years. Sometimes if you have a family history of colon cancer, you might need to be seen every five years.

Ms. Falade, it is important to me you get screened. Doing something is better than doing nothing. If you are adamant you do not want the colonoscopy, I can order the multitarget stool DNA test, which you can do at home and send to the lab. I did not initially offer this test to you because you were not sure what type of cancer your grandfather had. Usually, this test is not offered if you might be at high risk of getting colon cancer. Other screening tests you may consider are the flexible sigmoidoscopy, computed tomography colonography (virtual colonoscopy), a fecal immunochemical test (FIT), or the colon capsule. There is also the blood test called Septin 9, however it is not as good as the other tests which I mentioned.

If you have any questions, you can always call the office or send me your questions through the patient portal. For now, I will order the DNA test so it can be delivered to your home. Doing something is better than doing nothing.

Sincerely,

Ngozi Osuagwu, MD, FACOG

In the United States, colorectal cancer (CRC) is the third most common occurring cancer in both men and women.

Colonoscopy is the only one-step screening test. You can use this test to make a diagnosis and treat the problem.

All screening tests other than a colonoscopy are two-step tests.

Two-step tests require a colonoscopy if positive, to complete the screening process.

Shaukat, Aasma MD, MPH, FACG1,2; Kahi, Charles J. MD, MSc, FACG3,7; Burke, Carol A. MD, FACG4; Rabeneck, Linda MD, MPH, MACG5; Sauer, Bryan G. MD, MSc, FACG (GRADE Methodologist)6; Rex, Douglas K. MD, MACG3 ACG Clinical Guidelines: Colorectal Cancer Screening 2021, The American Journal of Gastroenterology: March 2021 - Volume 116 - Issue 3 - p 458-479 doi: 10.14309/ajg.0000000000001122

CONSTIPATION

Dear Ms. Lee,

At your appointment, you seemed surprised when I decided not to give you any medication. You have seen several physicians and they have told you that your lower abdominal pain was due to constipation. You have been given stool softeners and laxatives, which offered some relief. You mentioned relief for you is having a bowel movement every three days. Without the softener or laxative, you usually have one bowel movement per week. You often complain of feeling bloated and very uncomfortable.

After reviewing your history, the CT scan images and report, and performing a physical exam, I do agree with your previous physicians. You would benefit from having regular bowel movements. I believe you should have a bowel movement daily. Bowel movements allow us to remove the toxins from our body. It is hard for me to fathom that you are not eliminating daily.

The reason I did not write a prescription is because that would only be treating the symptom—we really need to figure out why you are constipated. You mentioned you hate drinking water. Keeping well hydrated is really important in helping with constipation. You need to increase your fluid intake. You might consider starting your day by drinking a full glass of room temperature water. Next, you need to increase the amount of fiber in your diet to about 25 grams of fiber per day. Foods that are rich in fiber include beans, fruits, vegetables, whole grains, and nuts. You should add fiber to your diet gradually to avoid feeling bloated. You might start by just eating oatmeal every day. Exercising is also important in having regular bowel movements. You have to be moving; I have found yoga to be very beneficial in terms of overall health and for maintaining regularity.

When you have the urge to have a bowel movement, have it. I know you mentioned you hate having a bowel movement at work; however, having a bowel movement is a natural part of life. You should not fight the urge.

I would also recommend that you see a gastroenterologist—a specialist who is an expert on the bowel. I prefer your primary care physician make that referral. If you have any further questions, please do not hesitate to contact me either by calling the office or via our online service using the special registration number you've received.

Sincerely,

Ngozi Osuagwu, MD, FACOG

Constipation is very common. Overall, approximately 16% of U.S. adults have symptoms of constipation, with approximately one-third of adults over 60 years of age reporting symptoms.

Source:American Gastroenterological Association, Bharucha AE, Dorn SD, Lembo A, Pressman A. American Gastroenterological Association medical position statement on constipation. Gastroenterology. 2013;144(1):211–217, https://www.gastrojournal.org/action/showPdf?pii=S0016-5085%2812%2901545-4(Accessed August 19, 2021).

HYPERTENSION

Dear Ms. Johnson

After you left the office, I spent some time reviewing your chart. You have been seeing me for the past four years. When you first visited my office, your blood pressure was 146/90. You told me your blood pressure had never been that high. You said it was the first time coming to my office and you were nervous. The following year, your blood pressure was 140/90. I asked you to speak with your primary care physician. You told me you would mention it to her. The next year, you told me that you had "a little bit of high blood pressure." I am still trying to figure out what that meant. Your primary care physician gave you medicine, but you felt you could get your blood pressure down if you exercised and lost weight. Today your blood pressure was 160/96.

Ms. Johnson, you are 45 years old. Your mother has high blood pressure. Your father died of a heart attack at age 50. You mentioned you thought that one of your grandparents had a stroke, but you were too young then to remember all the details. You have a family history of heart disease. You have high blood pressure. You need to be treated.

Ideally, the top number of your blood pressure, which is called the systolic blood pressure, should be less than 120, and the bottom number, which is called the diastolic blood pressure, should be less than 80. We do not tell you that you have high blood pressure, or hypertension, until we have checked your blood pressure more than twice and it is over 130/80. Sometimes, when the top number is between 120 and 140 and the bottom number is between 80 and 90, we start warning patients to really think about making lifestyle changes to help bring their pressure down. This includes changes in the diet. I often talk about the DASH diet. DASH is an acronym for dietary approaches to stop hypertension. We want you to increase your consumption of fruits and vegetables. You can find more information on the DASH diet by going online and typing "DASH diet" in the search engine.

In your case, you need to start that diet and you need to take the medication your primary care physician prescribed. The leading cause of death in women is heart disease. It is important that we get your blood pressure under control. Ms. Johnson, if your blood pressure is not controlled, even while taking your medication you can go blind, you can have a stroke, or you can develop kidney disease. High blood pressure is a risk factor for dementia. You can even drop dead. Your children cannot afford to lose their mother in any capacity. Imagine if you have a stroke and you cannot live the way you did yesterday. You might not be able to walk or talk. You might not have control of your bladder. Is that fair to the children or your husband when you can make changes now that might prevent you from having problems in the future? Take the medicine.

Ms. Johnson, not only do I want you to take the medicine, I also want you to buy a blood pressure monitor. Anyone who has high blood pressure should own a monitor. I have enclosed a prescription. Some insurance companies cover the cost of a monitor, but even if they do not pay for the monitor, it is a worthwhile investment. Once you get the monitor, I would like you to take your blood pressure twice a day and record it in a notebook. You can then share this information with your primary care physician, and it will tell your doctor if the medicine is working and whether she needs to make adjustments in the dosage, change the medication, or add an additional medication. Once your blood pressure is under control, you will only need to check it once a week.

Some medicines may have side effects such dry cough or decreased sex drive. If you experience side effects, do not stop taking your medication. Instead, talk to your doctor. There are hundreds of blood pressure medications; there will be a right one for you.

Ms. Johnson, I know that you have been reluctant to get on medication because you do not want to take medication for the rest of your life. Lifestyle changes are important. I believe if you follow the DASH diet, start exercising, and lose some weight, you might notice you do not need as much medication and you might one day be able to go off the medication. But right now, it is important to take your medication as prescribed.

I know that you came to me today because of vulvar itching, and you probably are asking what your blood pressure has to do with your itching. They are not related, but we do check your blood pressure at every visit. Regarding your itching, I believe it is an allergic reaction to the toilet paper you recently bought. Try going back to the old one you used to use and tell me if your symptoms resolve. I look forward to seeing you for your annual exam in six months.

Sincerely,

Ngozi Osuagwu, MD, FACOG

On average, someone dies of cardiovascular disease (CVD) every 36 seconds in the United States.

Approximately every 39 seconds, an American will have a heart attack. The average age of a first heart attack is 65.6 years old for men and 72.0 years old for women.

On average, someone in the United States has a stroke every 40 seconds. There are about 795,000 new or recurrent strokes each year.

On average, someone dies of a stroke every 3 minutes and 33 seconds in the United States. There are about 405 deaths from stroke each day.

About 47.3% of adults in the United States have high blood pressure.

You can reduce the risk of heart disease by following the American Heart Association's Life's Simple 7:

1. *Do not use any kind of tobacco products*

2. *Increase physical activity*

3. *Follow a heart-healthy diet*

4. *Maintain healthy body weight*

5. *Control cholesterol*

6. *Control blood pressure*

7. *Control blood sugar*

Source: Virani SS, Alonso, A, et al. Heart Disease and Stroke Statistics – 2021 Update: A Report from the American Heart Association. Circulation 2021; 143(8):e254–e743. https://www.ahajournals.org/doi/10.1161/CIR.0000000000000950 (Accessed August 18, 2021).

HEART ATTACK

Dear Ms. Daniels,

I am so happy to hear that you are feeling better. I saw your daughter and she told me what happened. She said you've had a rough three months, but you're doing better. I am so happy you listened to your body and went to the emergency room when you did. She said she was shocked to find out you had a heart attack. She said no one in your family had heart disease, so you were in shock as well. I am just so happy you are better. She said what finally made you call her was the jaw pain—you were actually upset with the dentist. You thought the dentist had done something while cleaning your teeth.

I know you were surprised because you never had chest pain. She said you had not been feeling very well throughout the day. You had some nausea and vomiting and thought it was because of what you ate at lunch. You were sweating and thought it was another hot flash. You just felt blah. When you called her, she insisted you take an aspirin and call the ambulance. Ms. Daniels, you had the classic signs of a heart attack; general malaise, sweating, nausea, and jaw pain are all signs in women. I know most people believe a heart attack should be associated with chest pain, and this is often the case; however with women, there may be other symptoms. Our symptoms are different from men's. Sometimes women may have chest pain, but they can also have the symptoms you described.

Your daughter also mentioned in the hospital your blood pressure was borderline high. Ms. Daniels, we have been talking about your blood pressure for years, but you told me it was "stress". I hope you will take your medications as prescribed. You are right stress may be a contributing factor, but while we are trying to manage the stress, you should continue to take your blood pressure medication.

I am also writing for another reason. It has been over three years since your last well woman exam. Let us work together to keep you healthy. Please call the office and schedule your appointment. Once again, I am glad that you are doing better, and I look forward to seeing you soon.

Sincerely,

Ngozi Osuagwu, MD, FACOG

Heart disease is the No. 1 killer of women in the United States.

If you have any of these signs, call 9-1-1 and get to the hospital right away:

+ *Uncomfortable pressure, squeezing, fullness, or pain in the center of the chest that lasts more than a few minutes or goes away and comes back*

+ *Pain or discomfort in one or both arms or the back, neck, jaw, or stomach*

+ *Shortness of breath with or without chest discomfort*

+ *Breaking out in a cold sweat, nausea, or lightheadedness*

+ *As with men, women's most common heart attack symptom is chest pain or discomfort; however, women are somewhat more likely than men to experience some of the other symptoms, particularly shortness of breath, nausea/vomiting, and back or jaw pain*

Source: American Heart Association. Heart Attack Symptoms in Women. https://www.heart.org/en/health-topics/heart-attack/ warning-signs-of-a-heart-attack/heart-attack-symptoms-in-women (Accessed August 18, 2021).

DECREASED LIBIDO

Dear Ari,

You mentioned you wanted to know more about the new medication that was approved for women with decreased libido. During your office visit you informed me you suffered from decreased libido and the inability to reach an orgasm.

There are actually two medications that are available. One of the drugs is called Flibanserin or Addyi and comes in a pill form. The other medication is Bremelanotide, or Vylessi, which you have to inject under the skin in the belly or thigh. Both are for premenopausal women who have low sexual desire that causes some distress. These medications cannot be used for women who have psychiatric problems or are using certain other medications. They are also not used for women who have problems with their relationships. I will not be prescribing either medication for you.

I know you also mentioned giving you testosterone to see if that will be helpful. Testosterone can help; however, there are no approved female testosterone products. For this reason, I am uncomfortable prescribing testosterone at this time.

Ari, I have known you for many years. You will not be able to have an increase in desire or reach an orgasm with someone that you do not love. There will never be a medication out there to help you with that. You need to fix your relationship or get out of it all together. I do not think it is healthy for you or your children.

Yes, the ideal thing would be to stay married forever. You mentioned you took your vows seriously, but you have to remember the initial reason you got married was because you were pregnant, and you felt it was the right thing to do. In the 10 years I have known you, you have never once told me that you loved your husband. Love is such an important part of marriage and is so important in maintaining a household. I know you have already gone to marriage counseling and it did not seem to work the way you expected.

Again, you have to make the decision. I know that this situation is affecting your health; you appear very anxious these days and your blood pressure is up. I am available if you need to talk. Please do not hesitate to schedule an appointment.

Sincerely,

Ngozi Osuagwu, MD, FACOG

According to the Prevalence of Female Sexual Problems Associated with Distress and Determinants of Treatment Seeking (PRESIDE) study, the prevalence of sexual dysfunction in U.S. women is 44%, though only 12% is associated with distress.

The most common type of sexual dysfunction reported in the study is low sexual desire.

The prevalence of sexual dysfunction is highest in women over the age of 65; however, this age group had the lowest prevalence of distress. The age group with the highest prevalence of distress is between 45 and 65 years old.

Source: Shifren JL, Monz BU, Russo PA, Segreti A, Johannes CB. Sexual Problems and Distress in the United States Women: Prevalence and Correlates. Obstet Gynecol 2008;112:970–978. https://journals.lww.com/greenjournal/fulltext/2008/11000/sexual_problems_and_distress_in_united_states.3.aspx (Accessed August 18, 2021)

OSTEOPOROSIS

Dear Ms. Woo,

I wanted to inform you central scheduling for the hospital will be calling you to schedule your bone density scan. I just received the report from the emergency room, and I am sorry to hear about the fall that led to the fracture of your wrist. I know you are upset you have to wear a cast for six weeks, but it will ensure that the fracture heals correctly and give us time to assess the health of your bones. I reviewed the report and your history and saw you mentioned your grandmother, mother, and maternal aunt had osteoporosis. I know you are only 49 years old, but because of the strong family history and this recent fracture, I believe you would benefit from a bone density scan to make sure you do not have low bone density or even osteoporosis.

I also know you have two daughters, and I think it would be great for you to share ways to help prevent osteoporosis with them. They are too young to get a bone density scan, but this is a perfect time to discuss prevention with them—waiting until they are your age to talk about it might be too late. Your primary risk factors are you are Asian and you are very thin. To help prevent osteoporosis, you must eat well and get the recommended amount of calcium and vitamin D. Since your daughters are under 50 years old, they should be getting at least 1000 mg of calcium and 400–800 IU of vitamin D per day. It is best to get calcium through your diet. Exposure to sunshine is the best way to get vitamin D; however, when the sun is not available, supplements usually provide enough vitamin D. Please encourage them to eat a well-balanced diet and to maintain a healthy weight.The next thing for them to do regularly is to exercise. Weight-bearing and strength exercise are best. Weight-bearing means any exercise where one is carrying their weight, like walking, dancing, jogging, or yoga. Additionally, since smoking and drinking excessive alcohol can contribute to osteoporosis, I would definitely emphasize not adding these bad habits.

Ms. Woo, what I mentioned is not only for your daughters, but also for you. Once you get the scan, please call the office to schedule an appointment for your annual exam. I can talk to you about the results at that time.

Sincerely,

Ngozi Osuagwu, MD, FACOG

Osteoporosis is a disease in which the bones become fragile and are likely to break. If not prevented or if left untreated, osteoporosis can progress painlessly until a bone breaks. The bones likely to break due to osteoporosis are located in the hip, spine, or wrist.

Osteoporosis is often called a silent disease because one can't feel bones weakening.

Approximately one in two women over the age of 50 will have an osteoporosis-related fracture in their remaining lifetime.

Osteoporosis may limit mobility, which often leads to feelings of isolation or depression. Additionally, 20 percent of seniors who break a hip die within one year from complications related to either the broken bone itself or the surgery to repair it. Many patients require long-term nursing home care.

Source: National Osteoporosis Foundation. *What is Osteoporosis and What Causes It?* https://www.nof.org/patients/what-is-osteoporosis/ (Accessed August 20, 2021).

POSTMENOPAUSAL WEIGHT MANAGEMENT

Dear Ms. Harden

I did not mean for you to leave my office feeling helpless. My intention was to make you feel better about yourself. You are 56 years old and have been overweight most of your life. You have told me you cannot remember a time in your life when you were not dieting. You mentioned you would go on a diet, lose weight, gain it back, and even add a few more pounds. You told me for the past two years, you have really tried to work out and eat right, yet nothing seems to be happening, and you feel there is nothing that you can do. You also shared since you became menopausal, it has been really difficult to lose weight— you have to practically stop eating just to lose weight, and that, of course, is impossible.

What a lot of women do not realize is that it is extremely difficult to lose weight once you reach menopause. Studies have shown your best bet to being at the weight you would like to be is to reach that weight before you are menopausal. I hate to go backward, but the amount of exercise and the lifestyle changes you have made over the past year, if it were done just a decade earlier, would have led to more weight loss. To lose weight after menopause, not only do the calories you ingest have to be markedly decreased, but you have to exercise 90 minutes a day for about six days a week. It is difficult but not necessarily impossible to keep up with that kind of regimen, especially if you were not doing it prior to menopause.

Here are your options: The first option is to maintain your current weight. I know that assumes you can live with your current weight. What you must realize is at menopause, weight maintenance is progress, because if you do nothing, you will gain weight. You will need to invest in a scale and place it in the bathroom. Getting on the scale daily will be part of your routine. You are 196 pounds. Let our goal be staying below 200 pounds. When you check your weight in the morning and you see 198 pounds, maybe that day you will just eat three meals and no dessert. You might even work out a little extra. If you step on the scale and you see 195 pounds, you can splurge a little on dessert. The purpose of checking your weight regularly is for you to have a sense of your weight, so you are less likely to get frustrated. You will never get on the scale and see a 10-pound weight gain, because you have been checking your weight regularly. I know this works, because I have been doing it for years. There is a National Weight Registry, which is an ongoing re-search project focusing on people who have lost weight and main-tained their weight loss for over a year. What the participants had in common was checking their weight regularly. They also suggest eating breakfast every day, exercising six days a week, eating a low-fat diet, and watching less than 10 hours per week of television.

The other option is to have surgery—bariatric surgery. I am not talking about liposuction or a tummy tuck, but surgery that chang-es your stomach. We can make the stomach smaller by removing part of it, or we can change the way food passes through your in-testine. If you choose this option, it will take about six months from the time you see the surgeon until you have the surgery. With bar-iatric surgery, you would be managed by a team. The team would include the surgeon as well as a dietician, an exercise trainer, and a psychologist. All these professionals want to make sure that you understand the commitment that is required to lose weight.

Only you can decide which of these options you choose. I just want you to stop beating up on yourself because you cannot lose weight. You are postmenopausal, and barring surgery, you are unlikely to lose a significant amount. I know that might seem pessimistic, but it is the truth. Let us enjoy life.

Right now, focus on how you feel. You told me when you work out you feel wonderful. So work out. You also said that when you eat fruits and vegetables, you tend to have more energy. So eat fruits and vegetables. Both of these will benefit your health, help you feel better, and at the very least help you maintain your current weight.

Please call the office if you have any other concerns. Take care.

Sincerely,

Ngozi Osuagwu, MD, FACOG

Obesity in the United States disproportionately affects women. In 2013 -2014 US age –adjusted prevalence of obesity (body mass index [BMI] at or above 30 kg/m2) was 40.4% in women compared with 35% in men.

Prevalence of severe obesity (BMI at or greater than 40 kg/m2) is nearly double in women (9.9%) compared with men (5.5%) and continues to increase.

Many women gain weight during the menopause transition.

Weight gain during menopause transition seems to be related mostly to aging and lifestyle.

Inadequate or disordered sleep is associated with obesity and weight gain.

Elevated BMI has been associated with more frequent or severe hot flashes.

Source: The North American Menopause Society (NAMS). Menopause Practice: A Clinician's Guide, 6th ed. Pepper Pike, OH: NAMS, 2019. 24 – 27.

ABNORMAL UTERINE BLEEDING

Dear Ms. Nowak,

I want to once again review the plan of action for your treatment. I know you have seen several physicians due to abnormal bleeding, and I want to be clear, I am not going to solve your problems in two to three visits. It might take a little while. I am also not going to string you along. You have to be patient. Once we figure out what is wrong, I can then treat you appropriately. I know you mentioned your friend had the intrauterine device (IUD) that contained hormones and she is doing well, but that might not be the best management option for you.

You are 46 years old and said for the past two years your periods have been irregular; you would sometimes skip a month, and when it did come it could last for a full month. Most of the time, your periods last for two weeks. The bleeding can be light, or sometimes it could be heavy. When it is heavy, you are passing large clots. You mentioned you have had several accidents at work, causing you to wear dark clothing since you do not know when the bleeding will occur, and that you are constantly changing your sheets at night. You said you have been taking iron tablets twice a day because you feel weak. You also mentioned your relationship with your husband is being affected because you do not feel comfortable having sex when you are bleeding. You stated to me that you feel like crap. I get it.

As I mentioned during the office visit, there are several reasons for abnormal bleeding. Abnormal bleeding can be caused by problems with your uterus or problems that are not related to the uterus. Problems with the uterus include polyps (abnormal tissue growths in the uterus), adenomyosis (when the tissue that lines the uterus is found in the muscle of the uterus), fibroids (benign growths of uterus; these are very common), precancer, or cancer. The problems that are not related to the uterus include problems with clotting, meaning that you do not have the ability to form clots, or problems ovulating. There are times when we finish doing the work-up and we cannot find a reason why a patient is bleeding abnormally. The good news with this is we have eliminated all the really bad reasons why you may have abnormal bleeding, then I can treat you.

You had blood work today. I drew a complete blood count (CBC) to check whether you are anemic and also to make sure you have clotting ability. I am also screening you for thyroid disease. You were not bleeding today, so I obtained a Pap smear with the human papillomavirus (HPV) test as well as cultures for gonorrhea, chlamydia, and trichomoniasis to make sure you do not have an infection. Finally, I ordered a pelvic ultrasound to check for fibroids and polyps. I will probably need to take a sample of your uterine lining to make sure that you do not have a precancerous lesion or cancer.

I am committed to finding out why you are bleeding this way. I look forward to seeing you at your next scheduled appointment to discuss your results and next steps. If you start to bleed before your appointment with me, please call the office and I will give you medicine to help with the bleeding until your appointment.

Sincerely,

Ngozi Osuagwu, MD, FACOG

Approximately one-third of women experience abnormal uterine bleeding at some time in their lives.

As many as half of affected women do not seek medical care, even if they have access to a healthcare provider.

Source: Munro MG, Critchley HO, Fraser IS. The two FIGO Systems for Normal and Abnormal Uterine Bleeding Symptoms and Classification of Causes of Abnormal Uterine Bleeding in the Reproductive Years: 2018 Revisions. Int J Gynecol Obstet 2018;143(3):393–408.

POSTMENOPAUSAL BLEEDING

Dear Ms. Singh,

I am truly sorry I was unable to see you today. I was running late because I had a delivery earlier in the morning, and I do not have to remind you that babies come when they want. My staff informed me you came in but left after an hour. They also mentioned you left the office without rescheduling your appointment. You still need the sonohysterogram that you were supposed to get today.

You are 57 years old and mentioned your last menstrual period was at age 53. At your well woman visit two weeks ago, you mentioned you noted some vaginal bleeding. You described it as spotting and felt I was making a mountain out of a molehill. As I mentioned to you at your visit, no amount of bleeding at your age is normal. You should not be bleeding at age 57 years old if you have not had a period for four years. At your age, once you have gone a full year without a period and then have bleeding, it is called postmenopausal bleeding.

The Pap smear and HPV test performed at your earlier visit were both negative. Due to the bleeding, I checked you for gonorrhea and chlamydia, both of which were also negative. An ultrasound was ordered a few days later and it showed your uterus was of normal size; however, the lining of the uterus was nine millimeters. For a woman your age that has not had a period for four years, the lining should be less than four millimeters. In younger woman, nine millimeters would be normal. Your ovaries looked normal.

We need to get a sample of the lining of the uterus for screening to make sure you do not have cancer. When I spoke to you on the phone, I gave you the option of going to the operating room and having a hysteroscopy or having a procedure in the office called a sonohysterogram. A hysteroscopy can be performed in the office, but we perform ours in the hospital since our office is attached to the hospital. A hysteroscopy is where I put a telescope through the vagina inside the uterus. I then look at the walls of the uterus. If I see something abnormal, I immediately get a biopsy (a small tissue sample). If I do not see anything, I will perform a dilatation and curettage (D & C). The sonohysterogram is performed in the office. The sonohysterogram is where I put a catheter (a small tube) into the uterus and then put an ultrasound probe into the vagina. I will then inject water through the small tube while performing an ultrasound. This will allow me to look at the lining of the uterus well to find out why it is thick. If the lining looks about the same all over, I can perform a biopsy in the office. If I see something like fibroids or a polyp, then you will need to have a hysteroscopy.

We need to make sure you do not have cancer. The major concern is endometrial cancer. We do not have a way to screen for endometrial cancer like we do for cervical cancer or breast cancer. To screen for cervical cancer, we get Pap smears. To screen for breast cancer, we get mammograms. For endometrial cancer, we must wait for symptoms to occur; the most common symptom is bleeding. The good news with endometrial cancer is that if we find it early, we can actually get rid of the cancer. We find it early by women reporting their symptoms right away.

Ms. Singh, I do not wish to alarm you. I am not saying you have cancer. Most people who have postmenopausal bleeding do not have cancer, but there is no way to find out unless we start the work-up. We need to get a sample of the tissue in the uterus.

I am sorry I was running late today; I wrote this letter because I do not want your anger to get in the way of getting care. You need to follow up with a gynecologist. I will have you come in as the first appointment of the day if you still want the sonohysterogram, or I can book you for the operating room to have the hysteroscopy. Please call the office with your decision so we can schedule the procedure.

Sincerely,

Ngozi Osuagwu, MD, FACOG

In postmenopausal women, abnormal uterine bleeding (AUB) is associated with endometrial cancer in 5% of patients and with endometrial hyperplasia, endometrial polyps, or other pathology of the endometrium in 20% of patients.

In about 50–70% of patients, no organic cause of bleeding is found, and the postmenopausal AUB is often attributed to endometrial or vaginal atrophy.

Source: The North American Menopause Society (NAMS). Menopause Practice: A Clinician's Guide, 6th ed. Pepper Pike, OH: NAMS, 2019. 217.

URINARY INCONTINENCE

Dear Ms. Andrews,

I can sense that you were a little upset when you left the office. You finally had the courage to talk about an issue that seems to have been bothering you for quite a while. Here is the problem: When you scheduled your appointment, you scheduled a well woman exam. At the start of the exam, I asked you if you had any problems and you told me everything was going well. I finished examining you, and we discussed routine health maintenance issues like exercise and healthy diet. Just as you were leaving, you mentioned you had been having issues with urination. You mentioned you had been embarrassed to talk about it, but it had become bothersome for you. You should never feel embarrassed to talk with your gynecologist. Unfortunately, urinary incontinence is not something that I can evaluate in five minutes. Such an evaluation requires me getting additional history from you and performing an additional exam. You mentioned that you had a friend who had surgery which resolved her issues, but this is not the case for every woman.

Urinary incontinence is the involuntary loss of urine. The cause can be divided into three broad categories: stress urinary incontinence (losing urine when you cough or sneeze), urge urinary incontinence (having the need to void and losing control of the urine before you get to a bathroom), and mixed urinary incontinence (combination of stress and urge). There are various causes of each, and depending on the cause, the treatment varies. It might not be as simple as the surgery your friend had.

I sent your urine for urinalysis and culture, and everything came back negative. You did not have any blood in the urine, and you did not have an infection. I have enclosed a questionnaire and a voiding diary for you to complete. This will help me figure out what type of incontinence you might have and whether there are changes you can make. For example, some women who drink a lot of caffeine have issues with their bladder, and sometimes the medications that one is taking may play a role.

In terms of treatment, it might not necessarily be surgery you need. You may be able to do well with medication. You may even benefit from physical therapy.

One thing I want you to know is you do not have to suffer in silence. I am quite confident that I will be able to find the cause of your urinary incontinence. If I am not able to, I can refer you to a urogynecologist. These are gynecologists who have done additional training to take care of women with bladder and pelvic area problems.

Please schedule a follow-up appointment. If you have any questions, do not hesitate to contact the office. If you decide to go straight to a urogynecologist, my office can make the referral. Whether you return for a follow-up with me or go directly to a specialist, it would still be beneficial to complete the questionnaire and the voiding diary attached to this letter prior to this return visit with whichever doctor you decide.

Sincerely,

Ngozi Osuagwu, MD, FACOG

Urinary incontinence is a common condition in women of all ages.

Approximate percentage of women in each age category who experience some involuntary urine loss:

✦ *25% of young women,*

✦ *44–57% of middle-aged and postmenopausal women, and*

✦ *75% of older women.*

Despite the prevalence of urinary incontinence, many women are hesitant to seek care or discuss their symptoms with a physician. In a survey of women in the United States, only 45% of women who reported at least weekly urine leakage sought care for their incontinence symptoms.

Source: American College of Obstetricians and Gynecologists. ACOG Practice Bulletin 155: Urinary Incontinence in Women. Obstet Gynecol 2015;126(5):e66–e81.

VULVOVAGINAL ATROPHY/ GENITOURINARY SYNDROME OF MENOPAUSE (GSM)

Dear Ms. Patel,

You should never feel embarrassed to talk with your physician about anything. I am your gynecologist, and there is not much you can say that I have not heard. As we get older, vaginal burning and dryness are common. Unlike hot flashes, which can get better with time, the vaginal symptoms only get worse if we do not take action. You do not have to live in misery. You are having symptoms that are affecting you, and the only way I can help you is if you talk to me.

It has been over three years since you have had a period. You are now menopausal. Your ovaries are no longer producing estrogen. Although we always hear about hot flashes and feeling moody, vaginal problems are also very common when it comes to menopause. The problem is everyone thinks they are the only one with the issue, and that is wrong. It is common to be irritated and to have itching. Sex can be painful. Some women have problems with their bladder. They may have burning on urination, go to the bathroom a lot, or wake up in the middle of the night to use the bathroom. They may get a lot of urinary tract infections. Some women have abnormal discharge and may also have light bleeding after intercourse. These symptoms are most likely due to genitourinary syndrome of menopause. In the past, we would call it vulvovaginal atrophy (VVA), but you are having symptoms related to the vulva, vagina, and bladder. VVA is a thinning of the vulva (external genitalia) and the vagina.

I will need to see you in the office to examine you. As a gynecologist, I need to make sure that the symptoms I mentioned earlier are not due to a skin disorder, vaginal infection, bladder infection, or cancer. Most likely, it is due to the genitourinary syndrome of menopause.

You mentioned over-the-counter vaginal lubricants used to work but lately have not been helpful. You also told me you have been trying to have sex because you heard it would help, but it is so painful you have given up. Sex is important in a relationship, and if you want to have sex, there is help. You do not have to give up having sex; you just have to be willing to talk about what is going on and really think about your options.

I know when you left the office, you were going to think about what we discussed. I want to review what we discussed in the office. When your ovaries were working, they were producing the hormone estrogen. Estrogen makes the wall of the vagina thick and causes the wall of the vagina to produce glycogen. The glycogen mixes with the normal bacteria that are in the vagina, called lactobacilli, to produce lactic acid. This lactic acid protects the vagina; it is what causes your vagina to be acidic. In order to thicken the wall of the vagina and to get the pH of your vagina back to normal, it is important to put estrogen back in the vagina.

I know that you have been reluctant to use estrogen because you are afraid of cancer. I cannot promise you that you will not get cancer. What I can tell you is the dose of estrogen used to treat your symptoms is extremely low and is placed directly in the vagina, not taken by mouth. The amount of estrogen is so low I do not believe it would increase your risk of developing cancer.

Estrogen for the vagina comes in a cream, tablet, suppository, or ring. It will be up to you to choose what form of estrogen you would prefer. Every woman is different. For some women the cream is messy; some women do not feel comfortable putting the tablet applicator in the vagina; some women have issues inserting a suppository; and there are other women who cannot imagine leaving anything like a ring in the vagina for three months at a time. I have samples of each type in the office I can show you. Sometimes it is easier to make a decision if you see each one. Whatever you decide to use, it can take up to three months before you really notice an effect.

Besides estrogen, there are two other medications that are specific for women who are having discomfort when having intercourse: Ospemifene and Prasterone vaginal. Both are non-estrogen medications. Ospemifene works by binding in the same area estrogen would bind in the vagina to make the vaginal wall thicker. You would take this medication by mouth. Prasterone vaginal is dehydroepiandrosterone (DHEA) and when inserted in the vagina, it is converted to estrogen and testosterone.

I want you to know your symptoms are not out of the ordinary and you do not have to feel miserable. If you are interested in any of the prescription medications, please call the office. You can schedule an appointment if you need more information, or you can call with a pharmacy number and your choice of treatment, and I will call in the prescription. If you choose to do this, I would like to see you in three months to make sure your symptoms are improving. Take care.

Sincerely,

Ngozi Osuagwu, MD, FACOG

Genitourinary syndrome of menopause (GSM) affects approximately 27% to 84% of postmenopausal women and can have significantly impair health, sexual function, and quality of life.

GSM is likely underdiagnosed and undertreated.

In contrast to vasomotor symptoms (VMS) that usually improve over time, GSM is generally progressive (gets worse) without effective therapy.

Source: The 2020 genitourinary syndrome of menopause position statement of The North American Menopause Society, Menopause: September 2020 - Volume 27 - Issue 9 - p 976-992 doi: 10.1097/GME.0000000000001609. https://www.menopause.org/docs/default-source/default-document-library/2020-gsm-ps.pdf (Accessed August 21, 2021).

RETIREMENT

Dear Ms. Ramirez,

It was exciting to hear about your plans to retire in the next year. I still think that you will be too young to be retiring at age 50; however, you have put in 30 years with your job, so I understand. I also know it has been very difficult raising your children as a single mom, so it is probably time to rest. The good news is by the time you retire, your last child will be out of college.

As part of your exam, I ran some routine tests, and I have enclosed a copy of your lab results. Your Pap smear and human papillomavirus (HPV) test were negative. Gonorrhea, chlamydia and trichomoniasis were also negative, as was your HIV test.

Since it had been over two years since you last saw your family doctor, I ordered additional lab work. Your blood count was normal. You are not anemic. Your lipid profile, which tests your cholesterol, also came back normal. Your TSH test, which is a screening test for thyroid disease, was also normal.

I also checked your hemoglobin A1c level and it came back at seven percent, which concerns me. This result alone would indicate that you have diabetes. We never like to diagnose anyone as diabetic based on one blood result, so I would recommend you have the lab work repeated with your family doctor. You mentioned your family doctor told you two years ago you had prediabetes and noted it was important for you to think about your diet and to consider losing weight; however, based on your last visit with me, you actually gained 10 pounds over the past year, and your BMI is 35, which is considered obese. In addition, your blood pressure was 130/84. In the past, high blood pressure was defined as 140/90 or above, however under the new blood pressure guidelines from the American College of Cardiology and the American Heart Association, 130/80 or above is considered to be high blood pressure. My preference would be to have your blood pressure lower than 120/80. Diet and weight management are important for preventing and controlling both diabetes and blood pressure, and I strongly suggest that you discuss this with your family doctor as well.

I know I cannot force you to see your family doctor, nor can I force you to exercise or be mindful of what you eat. It needs to come from you. You need to decide it is important for you to make a change.

You mentioned in your visit with me, the first thing you want to do when you retire is to go on a cruise. You have been saving money every month to not only go on the cruise but also go on some of the excursions. The question is whether you will need to be dealing with insulin or pills when you go on the cruise, whether you will have the energy to enjoy the excursions, and whether you will be able to walk onto the cruise ship or be wheelchair bound.

I am not saying you cannot use insulin on the cruise ship or a cruise ship does not make accommodations for people in a wheelchair, but in your case, you are different. You did not have diabetes as a child and are not accustomed to giving yourself insulin. You want to board the cruise ship the way you have been going to work for the past 30 years. You can make the lifestyle changes to prevent the consequences of not managing your health now.

I do not believe people think about what kind of health they would like to be in when they retire, and I think that should be part of everyone's retirement plan. You can save all the money you want, but if you cannot enjoy your money when you are not working, was it worth it? Preventing illnesses by monitoring your weight and diet is a good place to start. Obesity is the second leading cause of preventable illness in the United States. It is linked to high blood pressure as well as diabetes, both of which are concerns for you. Both of these conditions can create problems with your heart, causing you to be less able to enjoy a long, active retirement.

I want you to be at your best when you retire next year. Please schedule an appointment with your family doctor. Please be mindful of what you are eating. Consider increasing the amount of vegetables, whole grains, and fruits in your diet. Avoid all the processed food. Consider limiting the amount of meat you eat. Take time to sit down and chew your food—it really makes a difference. In terms of exercise, do what you enjoy. Anything is better than nothing. I know you love to dance. Dance in front of a mirror. Walk in the neighborhood. And finally, make sure you get enough sleep.

Once again, I am happy for your impending retirement, and I look forward to seeing you in a year. If you have any questions or need to be seen earlier, please do not hesitate to contact the office to schedule an appointment.

Sincerely,

Ngozi Osuagwu, MD, FACOG

Chronic diseases are the leading cause of death and disability in America.

Six in ten adults in the United States have a chronic disease.

Four in ten adults in the United States have two or more chronic diseases.

Chronic diseases include heart disease, cancer, chronic lung disease, stroke, Alzheimer's disease, diabetes, and chronic kidney disease.

Lifestyle risks for chronic disease include tobacco use, poor nutrition, lack of physical activity, and excessive alcohol use.

Source: Centers for Disease Control and Prevention's National Center for Chronic Disease Prevention and Health Promotion. Chronic Diseases in America. https://www.cdc.gov/chronicdisease/resources/infographic/chronic-diseases.htm (Accessed August 21, 2021).

WHAT IS WRONG WITH BEING NATURAL?

What is wrong with being natural?

What is wrong with being me?

I need him to see me as I am, not what I was.

I do not want to go through the changes to be the person I was not.

So I took off the weave.

I stopped wearing a bra.

I allowed the hair between my legs to grow and grow.

I did not use the mascara and I did not apply the eyeliner.

I took off the lashes.

If he loved me, he would have to love who I really am.

I stopped coloring my hair

The fake nails were gone.

Yes, he would see me for what I am, not what I was.

I needed to go natural

I needed to be me.

I needed to tell the world that I am beautiful as I am and not as I was.

INDEX

Page numbers in bold indicate tables.

L

M

W

Walking, 71, 140
Weight loss, 70, 142, 143
Weight management, 160
Withdrawal (birth control method), 56–57

Y

Yeast infection, 47, 95, 99
diabetes and, 92–93

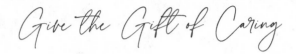

Give the Gift of Caring

This book is available at Amazon or Barnes and Nobles.
Copies of the book can also be purchased directly from the website:
http://www.ngoziosuagwumd.com

Phone Sales: **+1(614) 939-0595**
or write us at:
Ben Bosah Books, P O Box 671, New Albany, Ohio 43054.
Email address: BenBosahBooks@BenBosahBooks.com

Ben Bosah Books will make copies of Sincerely, Your Gynecologist
available at special quantity discounts for bulk purchases for sales
promotions, premiums, fund-raising, health fairs, or educational
use. Special books or books excerpts can also be created from
Sincerely, Your Gynecologist to suit specific requirements.

Dr. Ngozi Osuagwu is a sought after keynote speaker and can
add flavor to your events and conferences. Reach her via email at
drngozi@ngoziosuagwumd.com